UNDOCTORED

The Story of a Medic Who Ran Out of Patients

Adam Kay

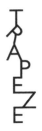

This book contains pregnancy loss, depictions of disordered eating behaviours, including methods, and details of sexual violence.

First published in Great Britain in 2022 by Trapeze,
an imprint of The Orion Publishing Group Ltd
Carmelite House, 50 Victoria Embankment
London EC4Y 0DZ

An Hachette UK Company

3 5 7 9 10 8 6 4

A CIP catalogue record for this book is
available from the British Library.

ISBN (Hardback) 978 1 39870 037 6
ISBN (Export Trade Paperback) 978 1 39870 038 3
ISBN (eBook) 978 1 39870 040 6
ISBN (Audio) 978 1 39870 041 3

Typeset by Input Data Services Ltd, Somerset

Printed in Great Britain by Clays Ltd, Elcograf S.p.A.

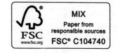

MIX
Paper from
responsible sources
FSC® C104740

www.orionbooks.co.uk

To Mike Schachter, for my GSOH.

And to my friends and family, who will once again learn quite major things about me by reading them in a book.

Disclaimer

Colleagues and friends have been anonymised in this book by replacing their names with members of the Marvel Cinematic Universe, an organisation which I'm pretty sure has no lawyers. Anonymising my family would have been harder, so I haven't bothered.

– FLASHBACK –

Formaldehyde

You know what it's like when you're cutting up a dead body. No, of course you don't. It's a perverse and horrific thing that should only ever be experienced by coroners and gangland criminals. Unless of course you're one of the 9,000 eighteen-year-olds who sign up to medical school in the UK every year. For them, it's just what you do each Friday morning.

'Wear your worst shirt and trousers,' advised a friendly second year before our first dissection.* 'Underwear too. Put on the same stuff every week, then burn it at the end of the year.' I imagined this was because they'd be getting sprayed with skull-water or stained by lung fragments, but it was actually around 2 per cent less disgusting than that – it was the stench.

The smell of the dissection room permeates deep into every single fibre of cotton or polyester and never, ever leaves. It hits you afresh whenever you're within 100 metres of the place: a smell I've never experienced since and one that isn't likely to trouble the parfumiers at Jo Malone any

---

* 'DISS-ection', as our anatomy lecturer taught us on day one: 'Diss as in piss, not dice as in lice.'

time soon. It's a weird blend of time-expired flesh and throat-grabbing, nose-scorching, eye-cooking industrial vinegar.

Two hundred of us paraded in, all pretending that what we were about to do was absolutely normal. Nervousness was overcompensated for by bullishness and laddishness. I called on behaviour I'd learned at countless hundred West Ham matches: just pretend to be one of them. Except, in this case, everyone there was pretending.*

'Find yourselves a cadaver,' bellowed our lecturer, like he was running the bingo night on a cruise ship.† We each huddled around one of the dozen zip-locked corpsebags.

'Do you mind if I join you?' I stuttered to my cadaver-mates, as if I was making up a four for bridge rather than getting ready to carve up someone's granddad like a Christmas turkey. Refusing to acknowledge our natural anxiety, we tried to outdo one another with how totally fine and comfortable we all felt. But despite our forced nonchalance, this was all palpably weird and disturbing. The scariest thing most of us had ever done at that point in our lives was mess around with a ouija board or com-petitively masturbate onto a biscuit.‡ And here we were, about to slice up a human being.

This sudden responsibility, a parachute-free plunge into the adult world, was quite the change for a voice-barely-broken, balls-barely-dropped teenager – like accidentally

---

* 'What?! You're a football fan?! This is the most explosive revelation in the entire book!' said my friend Justin.

† Sixty-three, septic knee.

‡ Much like when dunking in a mug of tea, I find the Rich Tea takes longest to disintegrate.

shifting the car into reverse when you're doing seventy on the M1.

Time to unzip the bag then.

First the face: waxy, yellowish, almost, but not quite, inhuman. Immediately some rugby jock called Thor quipped that he looked like Bruce Willis's nan and the rest of us laughed, desperate for some, any, emotional release. Then came the chest, unusually hairy. 'We've got a Wookiee!' another fresher whispered. Again we laughed, before wondering aloud whether chest hair keeps growing after death.* The abdomen was next, wrinkled like his organs were vacuum-packed inside. Then as the zip continued down and the PVC was peeled back, we all gasped. This man had an absolutely enormous penis.

Part of me felt like it was my turn to chip in with some light-hearted quip, just to show how totally unbothered I was by this immersive horror-movie experience. I couldn't – not yet, anyway. But nor did I object to the banter; showing compassion or respect would be opening myself up to ridicule. Week one and we were learning to fold and pack away our most human feelings.

There's really no reason to hack up a human in your first year, or indeed at all. There are better alternatives; models, 3D visualisations, even prosections, where you're shown a single autopsy by an expert rather than just barging in yourself like Teen Zorro. But instead, with freshers' week hangovers still pulsating behind our eyes, we were tossed

---

* It doesn't. Nor do your fingernails or toenails. Death involves every single cell of your body permanently signing off. It's pretty final like that. Instead, what people have probably noticed is that the skin around the nails and hair dries up, retracts and retreats, making it look like you need a postmortem mani-pedi.

in at the deep end with a scalpel and a licence to deal in dark humour. And let's not forget, we were teenagers, and there's no way a cock of that magnitude was going to escape unremarked upon.

'Does *that* grow after death too?' snorted one of my colleagues.* Another student gave it a flick and christened the dead guy Thundersword.† The ridiculousness of the male obsession with cock size engorges substantially when faced with a corpse. Of course, in reality, this gentleman's generous penis should be of no more interest or relevance than the corpse two tables down with big feet or long thumbs. Anyway, genitals were not the order of the day – our anatomy lecturer announced we were going to focus on the lungs. His instructions were quite simple: take one scalpel, take one corpse; make a nice straight line all the way down the breast bone, then turn it into an upside down T shape with a couple of slashes under the ribs. It won't bleed, he reminded us – our patients are dead, their hearts long past any pumping.

Although this was a new experience for all of us, as a lifelong vegetarian, I felt particularly ill-prepared. Everyone else around the table had been practising for this moment their entire lives by cutting into steaks and chicken breasts. The nearest I'd come was a nice taut mozzarella. I reached for a scalpel, keen not only to prove my suitability for medicine but hopefully to show some kind of instinctive proficiency with a blade. As I stood there, the scalpel's point millimetres from the skin, I learned as much about

---

* Now a consultant in respiratory medicine.

† Now a consultant radiologist.

4

my own physiology as I did this guy's anatomy. My sympathetic nervous system went into overdrive: the quickening of my pulse, the prickling secretion of sweat glands and a tremor in my muscles that showed clearly in the wobble of the blade. Then there was the sudden and wholly unexpected wave of famishing hunger that happens to be an unfortunate side effect of inhaling formaldehyde.

When it finally made contact, the scalpel slid through the skin like it was cutting wrapping paper. I guess it makes sense – you never see surgeons in hospital dramas sawing away at skin like they're doing woodwork. I pulled the scalpel down the breastbone, keeping the line as straight as I could, which was difficult with my hand still trembling like a leaf in a wind tunnel. As promised, there was no bleeding. This made the subject seem even less of a real human being, which I have to say felt like a positive: it steadied my hand and made it easier to chef him up. I reached the bottom of the sternum and swung a hard left round under the ribs. It was feeling easier – I could be cutting through PlayDoh or . . . Jesus! Suddenly, he started bleeding. Heavily. Everywhere. The bloke was alive!

Everyone gasped. Thor screamed. I was half-expecting the patient to sit bolt upright on the gurney like Frankenstein's monster and demand an apology for our disrespectful remarks about his dick, when I noticed that, in actual fact, he wasn't bleeding at all. I was. I'd accidentally sliced through my own thumb. I sheepishly handed over scalpel duties to the student on my left and instinctively stuffed my bleeding thumb into my mouth like the child I felt and, of course, still was. And this is how I can confirm that while the smell of formaldehyde may be an appetite stimulant, the taste of it very much isn't.

Chapter 1

I wasn't sleeping well.

I'd always slept very well as a doctor. I didn't sleep *much* and I slept in some odd places – hunched over the steering wheel of my car, curled up next to a filing cabinet, leaning against a storeroom wall like a horse – but I slept well. I guess my brain knew that napping opportunities were rare, so it was always able to press the shut-down button at a second's notice, until awoken by the next bleep or buzzer.

Ever since leaving medicine a few months earlier, I found myself routinely waking up at 3 a.m. from the exact same nightmare. Standing in that labour ward operating theatre. My eyes fogging over as I realise the baby I've been racing to save is dead, his tiny hands still and perfect. Trying and failing to place the stitches that might stop this woman from bleeding to death. The same brain that won't remember my online banking login details was quite happy to reconstruct and restage the most harrowing day of my life in microscopic detail. The moment the anaesthetist turns off the incongruously jolly radio station. The blood clotting in my shoes. Feeling my voice crack as I ask the scrub nurse for stitch after stitch after stitch after swab after swab after swab. The moment my consultant removes the patient's uterus and makes this blood-soaked nightmare her only experience of childbirth. The moment when I ask the ITU doctor if she's going to be OK and he won't answer me.

And then I'd jolt awake, covered in a cold lick of sweat, my heart pounding through every wet pore. The comedown would last for hours. In my worst moments, I was afraid to go to sleep because of what I knew was going to play out.

Waking up in emotional agony, covered in an emulsion of tears and perspiration isn't exactly attractive to a new partner, and me and J were still in the 'trying hard to impress' stage.★ Obviously I couldn't tell him about what I was going through in case he realised he'd taken on a defective model. Handily, it was easy enough to pretend everything was alright because our relationship was being conducted remotely. I was living with my parents – every thirty-year-old's dream, but the only option in between the catastrophe of my breakup with H and saving up for the deposit on a rented flat. J lived in Glasgow; we'd met on the internet at a time where it was less embarrassing to say you'd found your partner in prison or at an STI clinic, then sealed the deal when I braved the Megabus a few months later. For some reason, he didn't want to abandon his promising job as a junior TV producer and move 400 miles south to live with an itinerant former doctor who he'd met three times. But the distance meant that it was fairly easy to pretend I was fine and sane and normal – besides, I'd been pretending one way or another for most of my life.

Considerably less easy was being productive during the day when you've only slept for three hours at night. And I needed to be productive: I'd gone from a safe–but–underpaid career as

---

★ For example, I'd recently taken to shaving my balls. It doesn't matter how many years you've spent professionally honing your surgical skills, this will always be a very nervy operation.

a doctor to an unsafe-and-unpaid career as a writer-comedian. I was desperately willing comedy to work out. It was something I'd dabbled in over the years, both as a hobby and as an escape from the labour ward pressure-cooker, and I'd pretty much invested all of my hopes in it. Perhaps sucking me in the hardest was the fact that the stakes were so refreshingly low – there's no formal inquiry when a joke dies. But when you're a doctor, the jobs come to you: they knock on a clinic door or get pushed, screaming, into a labour ward. Writing jobs don't do that – you have to go and get them, which is tricky when you're living on a diet of Pro Plus and PTSD. But I needed to because otherwise . . . well, I didn't know what happened otherwise. This was my best attempt at a Plan B and there wasn't a Plan C. There was always the option of reversing back to Plan A, like so many quitter doctors before me. But the thought of revisiting medicine felt like returning to an abusive relationship.

No mealtime passed without a subtle hint from my parents that I should go back to medicine, usually something along the lines of, 'Why don't you go back to medicine?' or 'You're not even that funny, Adam.' I wasn't sure whether this was because they were worried about me, worried about what people might think about me or worried about what people might think of them. The thought did occur to me that if they'd left me to it in the first place, I might have found a job I was actually capable of. But that was never an option – being a doctor was preordained: much like Jesus, a boy pressured into his dad's line of work (miracles).

Medicine was revered in my household. It was the family trade – my dad was a mild-flavoured GP of forty years standing, with an enthusiasm for the job which didn't extend to

any other aspect of his life and couldn't fathom why, if you had the A levels, you wouldn't want to be a doctor too. There was an element of light snobbery – 'My son the doctor' could be referenced at book club and theatre club and lunch club.*
Why even have a child if you can't crow about their success? Plus, immigrant values take more than one generation to shake – our Polish DNA didn't just demand that we worked, they had to be the hardest, toughest jobs, rising as fast and as far as we could to show the country we'd earned our place. 'Light-hearted writer of goofs' wasn't an option on the forms my great-grandparents signed when they stepped off the boat, escaping Nazi persecution.

But career chat was slightly preferable to the other topic of conversation available – that I'd blown up my marriage to a woman (and a very nice woman at that) and was now in a relationship with a bloke (and a Scottish bloke at that). Everything in my life that had given me stability and them bragging rights – 'My son the straight doctor who sleeps comfortably through the night' – had been obliterated. Perhaps their little digs ('Why don't you put that in one of your skits?') were their coping mechanism, even if they weren't particularly helping me cope.

A couple of weeks into my stay, my dad announced he had a surprise for me. He announced it matter-of-factly, which led me to assume it wasn't going to be a chocolate eclair or a Labradoodle. He directed me up to the loft, where the entire roofspace was filled with hundreds upon hundreds of cardboard boxes. He gestured to a couple of ridges of the mountain. 'These ones are yours.'

---

* Whatever the fuck that is.

It turned out that over the previous three decades, totally unbeknown to me, my dad had collected every single piece of paper and every single object and artefact that had any connection whatsoever to me or my siblings. The accumulated bric-à-brac of four unfiltered human lives – every school exercise book, every terrible childhood drawing, every birthday or Christmas card, every piece of saxophone sheet music, every medical textbook, every crummy creation in Fimo or fusilli – all carefully boxed, labelled and hidden away in the loft.

It was particularly touching and surprising that a quiet man who had never to my knowledge expressed any degree of emotion whatsoever★ was secretly cataloguing every aspect of my existence. It must be said, he wasn't the most discriminating curator. Even if I'd grown up to be Shakespeare or Dolly Parton, no museum archive in the world would have been interested in my entrance ticket to the Derwent Pencil Museum.†

'Are you downsizing?' I asked.

'No', he replied. 'I'm just clearing out some of this crap.' His tone was slightly peeved, as if this unsolicited and borderline certifiable collection of memorabilia was somehow my responsibility, like a toddler I'd dropped off at his house and failed to pick up.

I spent a full week wading through this shanty town of

★ Forget the chicken and egg – does being a doctor extinguish your emotion or are the emotionless preternaturally drawn to the profession?

† You enter the Derwent Pencil Museum through a replica graphite mine. I always thought dying in a graphite mine would be a particularly embarrassing way to go out – risking life and limb so a schoolboy can scrawl a cock and balls onto their desk.

cardboard boxes. 'It's good you're occupying yourself while you decide what to do with your life,' said my mother, somehow forgetting the many times I had explained precisely what I was going to do with my life.

Several boxes were remnants of my time in medical school. As well as forests of long-forgotten lecture notes and metric tonnes of textbooks, there were also some more interesting relics.

My half-length white coat! As medical students, we were required to wear short versions of the classic white coat, so that senior doctors could identify us by sight and more easily humiliate us.

My first stethoscope! I tried it on for size and listened to my heart – the left ear wasn't working. Maybe it never had; I wouldn't have known back then.

My Evesham Micros Voyager 2000! A laptop with the weight, dimensions and processing power of a breeze block.

A poster for *AI: Artificial Insemination*! A piss-weak parody of a rightly forgotten Spielberg film, staged as the medical school's annual Soirée.

A couple of pots of nail polish! Christ, I must have been annoying.

A VHS tape from my slightly peculiar communication skills training!

My student ID card! It boasted the photo I initially provided the university: a spare photobooth snap I had from my passport renewal at age sixteen, which I didn't expect I'd be wearing pinned to my chest in hospitals a decade later because the university either couldn't or wouldn't update it.

And Dave! My half-skeleton.

For reasons that made little sense to me at the time and make even less sense to me now, medical students were encouraged to take possession of a large clattering boxful of actual human remains: a skull, vertebrae and various other orthopaedic essentials. I bought mine* from a student a few years ahead of me and named him Dave (after my beloved Duchovny). Much like anyone I brought back to my bedroom in those days, I had no idea what to do with him once he was there, so he just sat sulking creepily in the corner, like an emaciated emo teen.

I took his skull from the landfill of my past and held it in my right hand. Alas, poor Dave – I didn't know him at all. Had he consented to this particular afterlife? Did his surviving family have any idea that their great-great-grandfather's remains had been used and in some cases – let's not deny it – abused by an endless line of doctors-to-be? What was his job? Was he happy? Did he dance? Did he call it a bread roll or a bap? An entire life, right there in the palm of my hand.

I think, to my shame, this was probably the first time I'd given any thought to Dave's provenance. I also felt decidedly guilty that, however his before-life had treated him, his after-life must have been a grave disappointment: teaching me nothing about anatomy, then spending half a decade gathering dust in a loft with a bunch of report cards and ticket stubs. No, hang on – he did teach me something. He taught me how to juggle! I took out a humerus,† a femur and a tibia and gave them a few spins for old time's sake. Then, when they inevitably clattered to the floor, I paused.

How totally repulsive to juggle a dead man's bones. And

---

* If you're wondering how much a box of human remains cost, I paid £200 in 1998 for half a skeleton, which is about £350 today. Puts things in perspective, doesn't it? You've (hopefully) got one inside of you right now; it's the structure of your entire being – and it's barely worth a month's rent.

† I say that. It could have been anything from a fibula to a clavicle for all I knew.

doubly repulsive that it didn't bother me, that it felt . . . normal. That was actually what Dave had taught me; he'd performed the true function all skeletons must perform for their medical students. Just as time had stripped the flesh from his bones, he'd stripped the emotion from my perception of the human body – an essential skill, whether you're going to be making micrometre-accurate incisions in their cerebral artery or watching them die. The fact was, as well as teaching me to be a doctor, medical school changed me as a person, and not always for the better.

As a doctor, you can't get emotionally invested in every patient – you wouldn't be able to do your job – so an easy fix is not to get emotionally invested in any of them. In anything, really. Even if that means the odd bit of collateral damage – freezing out your partners who 'wouldn't understand', never speaking up about the toxicity you encounter, never opening up about your traumas. Even when they explode out of your subconscious and stop you from sleeping.

To be clear, I don't entirely blame medicine for how I turned out.

I also blame my parents.*

---

* I didn't really know what to do with Dave after rediscovering him. Putting him in the green bin with the organic waste didn't sit well with me ethically. Or legally, what with the Human Tissue Act 2004. In the end, I chucked him in the concrete footings of my parents' new patio, then phoned the police. Their parole date is 2042. (Or maybe I donated him to a medical school.)

Chapter 2

Steady your ball-shaving hand, grab yourself a helium heart, a box of perfumed truffles and a teddy bear which warbles 'I Will Always Love You' when you squeeze its thorax – it's Valentine's Day.

I'm in no danger of being overly sentimental – I've only been to Paris once (for a conference), and holding hands in the cinema is my romantic glass ceiling. Valentine's Day is fun by appointment – the romantic equivalent of a sales department's annual raft-building away day. A kind of virtual reality where baby-talk makes an unwelcome reappearance and spunking hard-earned cash on worthless tat that's pink, cock-shaped or made of chocolate (maybe even all three) is apparently mandatory.

There's something almost actively unpleasant about a restaurant on the 14th of February. It's a special occasion made entirely unspecial by fifty other couples at identical tables for two, eating an identical set menu with no deviations allowed (except for the £8 supplement for truffle shavings) and an identical undrinkably sweet Peppa Pig-coloured cocktail.

On the other hand, J had now got himself a job in London and the flat we were renting together was totally incompatible with a romantic dinner for two. The estate agent told us that we'd get used to the road noise, but it turns out that it was impossible to get used to the sound and vibration of the A40, transmitted through London's thinnest walls. On the plus side, when J caught me nightmaring awake in the early hours, I could always blame it on Eddie Stobart. But sweet nothings are better whispered than yelled, so we opted to eat out.

The (patriarchal, heteronormative) rule of the man organising the table for the Valentine's Day meal slightly breaks down in a gay relationship. I took the lead and booked this – our first Valentine's Day – and suggested we take it in turns afterwards. It showed confidence that I imagined many Valentine's dinners stretching before us. It also allowed me to choose somewhere vaguely affordable – my finances meant I felt my aorta tighten every time a direct debit left my account. And so it was that we ate in a busy but charmless restaurant with all the romantic ambience of a veterinary autopsy.

MENU
Starter: Smoked salmon with foam of beetroot and horseradish
Main: Heart-shaped steak with rosemary fries and asparagus

I mentioned to the waiter that I was vegetarian and he looked at me like I'd just ordered the sommelier, slow cooked, nose to tail. He agreed to speak to the chef and try to work something out.

VEGETARIAN MENU
Starter: Foam of beetroot and horseradish
Main: Rosemary fries and asparagus

Having found the big plate of foam funny, J was furious about my main. I told him it was actually fine and I wasn't that hungry anyway, having been professionally trained not to make a fuss.

Never one for tolerating an injustice, J was onto the waiter like a wolf on a panini.* Ten minutes later, the rosemary fries and asparagus returned, looking tired and emotional from their ping-pong shuttling, but this time garnished with a sad-looking fried egg. I immediately said, 'That looks perfect, thanks!' to prevent J from exploding.†

J suggested we salvage the evening by ordering a glass of champagne.

'Each?' I asked, nervous at the prospect of seeming miserly or unromantic, but more so at the prospect of not being able to afford anything else to eat for the rest of the month. J laughed, assuming I was trying out new material, and had the waiter bring two glasses of house fizz. I sipped it slowly, as if I was seven hours from a toilet break.

As we ate dessert (mine happily hadn't been replaced with a bowl of sawdust or a carburettor), I spotted Henry McCoy

---

* There was a long and fairly spirited discussion with my editor as to whether or not this metaphor worked. Whether, in fact, a wolf would go berserk for a panini. But it's my book and I maintain they would sprint across fields for them, laying waste to every Caffè Nero in sight.

† Sadly, this wasn't the worst Valentine's Day meal I would ever have. That accolade goes to one of J's subsequent choices, called 'Sky Suppers' or 'Pie in the Sky' or some such thing. A couple of dozen diners sit around a big square table in a carpark. The kitchen is in the middle of the table. Guests are then strapped into their seats with fighter-pilot seatbelts as a crane hoists the table a hundred feet into the air, where it wobbles around for a couple of hours as you eat a three-course dinner. Enjoyment of the meal depends entirely on diners being OK with heights, which I am not. I hadn't mentioned my fear of heights to J, of course, as I was still pretending to be at least partially sane. Even though it made no logical sense, I only felt safe up there if I had both hands firmly gripping the edge of the table. And so I did, for the duration of the evening, eating my dinner by lowering my face onto my plate like a cat.

on the other side of the dining room. He was a senior registrar I'd worked with a few years previously and the first person I'd encountered from my old life since I hobbled away from medicine. My brain played tricks on me, dressing him in scrubs before I blinked him back into his checked shirt. Napkins transformed into swabs, the smell of cooking meat became theatre diathermy. Ghosts from the ward were letting me know I wasn't quite free of them yet.

J asked if I was OK. I pointed Henry out to him and ran through some of his greatest hits: he'd once somehow caught a baby that his SHO had managed to drop mid-delivery,* he always brought a mini-scooter to work on nightshifts to speed up the endless walks from labour ward to A&E and he'd missed out on a research job because he crashed his Citroën Saxo into the BMW of a consultant who never forgave him.

I didn't recognise his Valentine but she definitely wasn't the same wife he'd had when we worked together. That was nearly five years earlier, though, which felt about right for medical spouse-churn – you're going to be hard pushed to watch two consecutive World Cups with the same partner if you're a doctor.

He spotted me as he was leaving (holding a single rose sheathed in cellophane – £8 supplement) and they trotted over. The WAGs introduced themselves and I marvelled, not for the first time, at how easily J struck up a conversation, asking the right questions, complimenting her on her pashmina, and how naturally she warmed to him. Meanwhile, Henry was asking me how I was doing in the tone not of an old colleague but in

---

* Maybe this is why medical schools insist on applicants being junior sports stars – you never know when you might need a wicket keeper.

the kind of voice you might reserve for a bereaved relative at a cremation.

I told him I was fine and jauntily pretended that writing was going very well indeed, thank you. He looked about as convinced as my mother. Which was when I found out that, apparently, by all accounts, I'd 'had a nervous breakdown'. This was news to me. I thought that I had walked away from a job I wasn't cut out for before it did me any more damage. The way McCoy was talking, the rumour mill had seen me carried off the premises ranting and gnashing then hurled into a padded cell. I guess it wasn't surprising. To a doctor, admitting that medicine isn't for you, that you can't hack it, is unthinkable, something only an unreasonable, out-of-control person would say out loud. Perhaps pathologising my departure was a way for them to avoid resenting me for escaping.*

The bill arrived and I was relieved to see J already had his card out and was silently waving away my – admittedly glacial – move to get my wallet. I bet McCoy barely flinched at his bill – a perk of the stable salary I threw away. As the waiter hovered with the card machine, Henry plus one said

---

* When I began gently testing the water about leaving the job, I was met with an onslaught of resistance, from faux concern all the way up to out-and-out guilt-tripping. Medicine was harder to leave than O2 or Virgin Active Gyms.

'You'll regret it.'

'You're nearly a consultant.'

'It'll be disastrous for your pension.'

It didn't seem to matter whether or not they knew about the nightmarish shift that broke me. They'd just chuck in some platitude about getting back on the horse, ignoring the fact that the horse in question had just trampled my internal organs to a steak tartare.

When I did eventually push the ejector seat button, I was so worried about what people might say that I left with barely a word. I informed the payroll people and my training director, and then I snuck out silently, a eunuch leaving an orgy.

their 'lovely to see you's and left. I could sense his fingers getting ready to text 'Guess who's gay?' around the hospitals of West London.

When J asked what we'd been talking about, I lied and said we were just reminiscing about the good old days.

– FLASHBACK –

The Good Old Days

Professor Stark was a perfect sphere – you could have hollowed him out and gone zorbing in him. He wore a pinstriped suit and a Union Jack bow-tie, before the days when wearing a Union Jack bow-tie meant nobody dared say the word 'refugee' in front of you. These were simpler times, when it merely meant that everyone referred to you behind your back as 'that weirdo in the bow-tie'.

He was a bowel surgeon who liked to think he was best known for his pioneering research on anastomosis of the large intestine, but in actual fact he was far better known for the time he asked a junior doctor assisting him in an operation to 'retract the gut'. Rather than take a metal retractor and move some bowel out of the operative field, the hapless junior used both of his hands to heave Prof Stark's stomach off to the side.

Our attachment with Prof Stark began on a Monday morning at the unpalatable hour of half past seven, when me and six other students filed into his office like America's Next Top Models and introduced ourselves. He called male medical students by their surnames and female medical students by their first names, for reasons of sexism. Except for Shakti, who he announced he was going to call Susan, for reasons of racism. Shakti didn't say any-thing and, shamefully, nor did anyone else. We might have been new to gastroenterology but we were old hands at shuttingthefuckupology. Medical students should be seen and not heard.★

At the end, he asked me to stay behind so he could have a few words, which were as follows: 'Get your hair cut. You look like a girl.'

I didn't look like a girl. And even if I did, Prof Stark could go fuck himself. My blond frosted tips – which pre-dated Facebook and therefore defy the existence of evidence to the contrary – looked fantastic.† My first thought was to stab him straight through the neck with the letter-opener on his desk, but in the end I went with my second thought of apologising profusely and saying I'd get it sorted at the weekend. He told me to get it sorted within the hour or I'd fail the attachment.

'It's eight in the morning,' I protested.

'It's a hospital – I'm sure even you can find a blade.'

Much as you wouldn't ask your barber to perform a quick hemicolectomy, medics don't make natural hairdressers.‡ I certainly didn't, in the outpatient block toilets with ban-dage scissors, my vision blurred by tears of powerlessness.

★ Antisemitism seemed fairly thin on the ground, which was . . . something? On one ward round, a different consultant described the antibiotic co-amoxiclav as being as popular among medics as a 'free bagel at a bar mitzvah'. A brave registrar pointed out to him that I was Jewish, to which the consultant informed him that I didn't mind, did I?

† I have since found my Young Person's Railcard, which unfortunately demon-strates that I actually looked like a waxwork model of Justin Timberlake shortly after it had been pulled from a particularly devastating fire.

‡ Just ask my scrotum.

'See, that looks much better,' Prof Stark announced when he saw me that afternoon. I looked like I'd just escaped from Rikers Island.

A big part of medical school training is about learning to fit in – or rather, learning to deal with being forced to fit in. Individuals turn up in the first year from all corners of the UK and beyond with a panoply of accents but, by the time they qualify, they share a single doctor-voice: beige, homogenous, acceptable. Any sartorial flare, individuality or artistic sensibility is similarly disappeared until you're all dressed like credit controllers or advertising a particularly sensible range of Debenhams workwear.*

As well as aesthetically distressing, this enforced homogenisation felt instinctively wrong. Why shouldn't we retain some individuality? Later that week, with all the doomed heroism of someone who's lived in the real world for the time it takes to soft-boil a quail's egg, I spoke to my educational supervisor to express my concerns. She sympathised but was realistic. 'Do you really want to take this anywhere?' She explained the uncomfortable lesson that being a troublemaker is possibly the worst reputation you can end up with in medicine. 'Who do you think is going to get booted out – him or you?'

---

* This mostly took place through slow, chronic learned behaviours and the occasional word from a consultant, but every now and then it found its way into official advice. In 2012 a, thankfully not NHS-sanctioned, guide to passing clinical exams was published by a senior GP, which advised candidates from Asia and Africa to switch to Scottish or Welsh accents instead, female candidates not to wear overly feminine dresses in case they looked too much like nurses, and for gay candidates to make sure their mannerisms, gait and speech weren't 'too overtly gay'.

And she was right, of course: what right-minded student would torpedo their future for the sake of a hairdo that makes them look like a nineties TV zookeeper? Reluctant to jet-wash my personality away entirely, I channelled my rebellion into micro-flamboyances, such as a single painted thumbnail. Large enough to symbolise a stand for self-expression, small enough to clench behind fingers or tuck away in a pocket when the dinosaurs were marching by. Personally, I couldn't see the problem with a little personality. Surely patients prefer doctors who are real people, individuals, like they are? You can get full marks in your written exams, but if you can't make a genuine connection with your patients then you're bullshit at your job.

Every Tuesday and Thursday morning we would forgo our leisurely 7.30 a.m. starts and haul ourselves in for 6 a.m. to review the patients on Prof's morning operating list. Patient JV was a guy in his early twenties, in for an anal fissure repair and the removal of a couple of polyps. He was extremely nervous. His level of anxiety – radiating off him like static electricity – was totally out of keeping with the scale of his operation, which was relatively minor, and certainly the smallest procedure Prof would be performing that day.

After I'd exhausted my list of standard questions, I tried to find out what was chewing him up. It's rare that a medical student can ever help a patient using their knowledge, but the one thing students have and doctors don't is time. I asked if anything was troubling him, if there was something he wanted to ask. There wasn't. I asked if he was worried about anything in particular. He wasn't. I asked him if he was worried that he might die during the operation. Not that either. Then I noticed him staring at my thumb.

'Am I . . . going to be able to have sex again?' he asked. I reassured him that yes, he absolutely would be able to have sex again and I'd find out from one of the doctors how long after the operation it would be. I could see every muscle of his body relax and I went off to the theatre staff room to get him his answer. It's a real buzz knowing that you've helped a patient – truly the best thing about the job, and the reason medics keep going – and that was the first time I'd felt it. And it was all (probably) thanks to a badly applied slick of mauve Superdrug nail polish.

Once Prof Stark's coterie of registrars had finished fake-laughing at one of his tired jokes, I jumped in. 'Prof, sorry to bother you. Patient JV – second on your list today. I was wondering if you could answer a quick question? How long after surgery will he be able to have . . . umm . . . anoreceptive intercourse?'

He mulled for a moment. 'Well, I'd probably wait till he's fully recovered from the anaesthetic if I were you.' The registrars roared with laughter and I turned pillar-box red.

Prof Stark pointed at my thumbnail. 'That had better be a bruise.'*

---

* The lawyers wouldn't allow me to use his actual name, but I really, really wanted to. Find me at a book signing and I'll probably just tell you: slander is much harder to prove than libel.

Chapter 3

How bad do you let something get before you bother your doctor? How long does your eye have to twitch and itch? A day? A week? Till it turns red? Till your eyeball slowly cracks apart and fifteen thousand maggots scrabble frantically over your cheeks? Not even then?

Some people pitch up at A&E convinced their bunion is early proof of the plague, while others will happily splint a compound fracture of their spine with a length of 4x2 and some fencing pins. Huge marketing campaigns do their best to educate the public about the signs and symptoms of heart attacks, but people will always call out an ambulance for a splash of diarrhoea, and all the billboards in the world won't change that. Popular culture also plays its part in miseducating the masses – that's why you're more likely to seek advice for a bleeding ear (because that's what happens to the baddie in films before he dies) than you are for a bleeding rectum (which only happens in more . . . niche movies). So metastasising bowel cancers often stay at home while every single perforated eardrum heads to A&E within moments. But you can't teach everyone everything, short of sending the entire population to medical school.*

---

* Which would admittedly solve the NHS staffing crisis.

Not that going to medical school makes you any better a patient. Doctors avoid going to see doctors. It's like a mechanic taking his car to another mechanic. It's embarrassing. You're always terrified you'll have your own diagnosis laughed out of the surgery. 'That's not a brain tumour – your hat's just too tight!'

Should my GP read this he'll be slightly alarmed to find out that during my time as a doctor, I took a regular Ventolin inhaler for asthma and gobbled numerous courses of self-prescribed antibiotics for respiratory tract infections and a bout of chlamydia.* Not ideal and not something the GMC would be too thrilled about, but still, a combination of medical knowledge and sheer luck kept me from doing any serious harm every time. Well, almost every time.

I was a year out of medicine and on my first holiday with J. To say I needed a break was an understatement: I was totally worn out from a post-medicine comedown which had the half-life of uranium. In the immediate fall-out, I hadn't exactly been in the holiday mood, even if we'd had the cash. We still didn't. We were only able to go abroad because a Louboutin-heeled friend of J's had paid for a trip we couldn't possibly have afforded as part of their fortieth birthday celebrations.

When somebody else is paying, you can find yourself in places you'd never dreamed of. Which is how I ended up staying at the Trump International Hotel in Las Vegas. Writing those words now, it's basically like announcing that I spent a fortnight in the Hitler Hilton, but back then Trump was just a slightly creepy reality-star-slash-business-bastard.

There's nothing quite like staying in a hotel owned by a

---

* Even if I'd wanted to see him, I'd have never got the time off work. To be honest, I'm surprised I had the time to catch chlamydia.

billionaire★ to make you realise how meagre your own cash reserves are. While the accommodation was paid for, we had to stump up spending money and Vegas is a city that just loves to relieve you of it. Every wedge salad or quart of unexceptional milkshake felt as if it was draining the budget for actual useful things we needed at home. Like electricity. At the rate we were going through those unhelpfully identical banknotes, we'd be living on uncooked toast the rest of the year. Thanks to a permanent state of financial anxiety, along with my usual insomnia and the pulverising grip of jet lag, it wasn't quite the relaxing, carefree vibe I'd been hoping for. Instead, I was a zombie who was too knackered to eat your brains. A wolf too tired to eat his panini.

On the third morning of the holiday, as I sauntered casually down the corridor of the thirty-fifth floor, my right leg completely stopped working and I collapsed into the (antiqued-gold effect) wall, then crumpled onto the (monogrammed, purple plush) carpet.

Hello illness, my old friend. My first personal medical emergency. I'd often wondered what might finally get me on that speeding gurney. Airlifted to hospital after a sleep-deprived car crash, perhaps? Losing a digit to a power tool? I hadn't reckoned on something as inexplicable, weird, unglamorous and utterly terrifying as random paralysis.

But this wasn't my debut at the rodeo, merely a new horse. Why should my approach be any different from the thousands of other medical emergencies I'd dealt with? That said, there were a few tiny differences: ordinarily I'd be dealing with a pregnant woman and J wouldn't be standing next to me,

★ Or so he claims.

clutching his face and appealing to various deities. Plus the patient wouldn't usually be me. Still, my technique would be exactly the same: stay calm, be methodical.*

First on the list, I despatched J to reception to see if they had a wheelchair we could borrow. This was primarily so that I could assess the situation in silence, without his frankly un-helpful yelling. I could move my hip, which was a good sign – my dance floor days weren't quite over. However, I couldn't move my right knee, ankle or foot, so I was unlikely to place that highly in the World Dance Olympiad. OK. So this prob-ably meant that something was pressing on some spinal nerve or other, and the things that do that are a) protruding discs or b) hideous, rampaging tumours. Calm, calm. The onset was a little too quick to be cancer, surely?†

Besides, my time as a doctor had drilled it into me that 'common things are common'. It sounds like something Dr Seuss would come up with after a night on the absinthe, but it's one of the most important rules in the medical game. Never ignore the possibility of the rare/dangerous/exciting diagnosis, but never forget that whatever's wrong with you is much more likely to be something relatively humdrum.

The vast majority of patients in this scenario – be they slumped in the gilded hallway of a prospective despot, or bent double in a pool of urine in Whitechapel station – wouldn't have cancer, and that included me. Fine. I calmly deduced it

---

* The old adage about the importance of doctors keeping their cool while they attend emergencies goes 'the first pulse you check is your own'. This is also liter-ally true when you're both the doctor and the patient.

† In nineties classic *Muriel's Wedding*, the character Rhonda suddenly collapses because of, it transpires, a paralysing tumour in her spine. Luckily that wasn't my inflight movie on the way over. Sorry, spoiler alert.

was a disc issue, which at the very worst would mean a fairly straightforward operation, but one with significant recuperation time. I reasoned therefore – it being only the third day of our holiday – that it couldn't do any harm to delay the surgery, so I decided to press on and enjoy myself as much as possible. My body could wait till we got home.

When J eventually returned with my wheelchair,★ however, he was rather insistent we call an ambulance. This was understandable, given I was splayed on the carpet like a chalk outline in *Bergerac*. Calling on my best 'Trust me, I'm a doctor' voice – patronising and pacifying patients for over a decade – I dismissed his concerns with a cheery wave from the carpet and promised him it was nothing that couldn't wait nine more days, when we were safely on the other side of the Gatwick Express. I didn't want to spend a single minute of my holiday in hospital, nor could I actually afford even half of a single minute of American healthcare. Besides, I'd vowed not to set foot in a hospital again when I handed in my badge and gun, and I was happy for that to include being a patient.

I spent the rest of the trip being pushed grumpily up and down the Strip, playing Blanche to J's increasingly resentful Baby Jane. Some positives in an otherwise shit-poor holiday: we got to skip the queue at every global buffet and craps table and even found ourselves upgraded to front-row seats for Elton John, where we had the honour of being soaked from head to foot in the great man's spit and sweat. (Unlike at Seaworld, no one hands out disposable ponchos.)

★ Vegas hotels are, I would say, suspiciously well-equipped for people collapsing in their corridors.

At the risk of sounding like one of those journalists who spends a week eking out a tenner before writing at length about the horrors of life on the breadline from their orangery, my temporary foray into wheelchair use was a genuine eye-opener. A holiday spent staring into the crotches of strangers meant I had plenty of time to make the following observations:

1. I have the upper-body strength of a hatchling sparrow and could only propel myself unaided at an agonising speed, and with agonising consequences for every bone and muscle in my arms.

2. A lot of people deemed it appropriate to ask what was wrong with me. ('So, how come you're in the chair, buddy?' 'I've got this condition which makes me tell you to go fuck yourself. Buddy.')

3. Even more people simply didn't bother talking to me at all and deferred to J, assuming I was mentally incapable of responding, sometimes even when I was the one who'd initiated the conversation.

4. Tables are the wrong height.

5. Mirrors are the wrong height.

6. Rolling through dog shit is extremely annoying.

Even though the rational, clear-headed medic in me was sure it was a disc, which would hopefully wiggle itself back into a less paralysing position with a bit of physio, the emotional, panicking patient in me couldn't shake the idea that it might be something more sinister. This wasn't helped by J constantly trying to find out what I wanted to happen after my death with all the subtlety of a rhino at the Ritz. 'Are there any songs that are particularly special to you?' 'Have you got any favourite charities?' 'When someone's partner dies, what's an acceptable number of weeks, sorry months, before they can start dating again?'*

I wasn't amazingly keen to head back into a hospital for any reason, but it didn't feel like there was much of an option, so I texted my friend Wilson to book myself an urgent MRI at his hospital for my return. There aren't a huge number of perks to being a doctor, but getting looked after by your colleagues is definitely one of them. Even when you've finished active duty you're still considered one of the club, and Wilson happily obliged. Then I cancelled it – of course it wasn't a tumour, I was being hysterical. What would I say to a patient who was convinced that their hangnail was a subungual melanoma and that death was mere seconds away? All I had to do was check in with my GP once we'd left the land of the not-so-free, like a normal person. Hang on, though, I'd already lost a few days by insisting we stay on holiday. How fast do tumours grow? I rebooked it. J cries at weddings of people he barely knows. How was he going to cope with a eulogy? Then I cancelled it again. By the time the two warring factions of my brain had reached a ceasefire and I re-rebooked the appointment for the final time, Wilson was almost certainly wishing a whole sackful of tumours on me.

Within forty-eight hours of landing in London, I was in an MRI waiting room, wearing one of those gowns designed by someone who likes staring at patients' bums. At first, there was something almost soothing about the familiarity of the hospital;

---

* A month for every year of the relationship plus three.

it wasn't one I'd ever worked in, but it might as well have been. The same smell and posters and bustle and automatic doors and distant alarms. And then I had this sudden unsettling feeling that someone was going to hand me a set of scrubs and a scalpel and send me off to do a caesarean section. My hands became clammy, the light was too bright, I struggled to swallow my saliva. I half-wanted to tear off the gown and run naked out of the nearest fire exit – although admittedly that might have added weight to the idea I'd had a breakdown.

Deep breath. I looked around the room for distractions. How weird to be sat on a chair in a waiting room, rather than kneeling down in front of a patient. Like waking up in bed with an ex you left years ago. I began to calm myself by leafing through a long printed menu of all the music available to listen to during the hour or so I'd be inside the scanner. It wasn't a great selection – the audio equivalent of the magazines in a dentist's waiting room – but, figuring something soothing would be appropriate, I plumped for Enya.

Before I knew it, I was being slid into the MRI machine like a chicken escalope into a George Foreman grill, headphones clamped to my ears and the instruction to stay perfectly still or the scan would be ruined. After a minute or so of managing not to sway rhythmically to the swelling Irish muzak, the MRI kicked in. I'm pretty sure I've never heard a louder noise in my life – it was like sharing a tumble-drier with a load of bricks while the sound of a thousand dial-up modems was piped directly into my brain. On the plus side, I didn't hear a second more Enya.

In order to remain perfectly still for an hour – crucial if you're to avoid your scan looking like a courtroom sketch drawn on a rollercoaster – I focused on a small heart scribbled in what was either felt tip or blood just inside the entrance of the MRI doughnut. How did it get there? Had someone graffitied inside the scanner? Had they brought a pen along especially? Had they done it during the scan itself? Or – equally possible – was I merely imagining it? I wouldn't be surprised if my nervous system was playing tricks on me, what with the tapestry of tumours I clearly . . . stop it. I must have sent thousands of patients down to radiology – 'Let's just do a quick scan of that' – and never once thought that I was sentencing them to an hour in silence with their own doom-laden thoughts. As unworkable as it might be logistically, there's an argument that every medical student should have a go at being a patient before they're allowed to qualify as a doctor.* Perhaps a quick hammer to the kneecap at the end of your first year followed by a week spent ignored on the ward might put you more in the patient's slippers than being taught to say 'That must be very difficult for you' in a communications skills module.

Me and J sat with the neurosurgeon as he pulled up my scans on his computer. He tapped with a pen on the screen like a weatherman at the end of his shift. 'Right, so you can see where this disc is protruding?'

I was saved! I squeezed J's thigh with delight and relief. He looked at me strangely, perhaps wondering why I was quite so delighted and relieved when I'd continually told him there was nothing to worry about. All my fears had been password-protected and locked away under layers of security: cancer, death, the awful arguments my mother and J would have at my wake ('Well, I didn't think he was that funny'). The surgeon kept tapping and pointing, using a lot of technical language that I didn't quite understand, presumably because he'd seen on my notes that I was a doctor.

---

* See also: everyone should have to spend a three-month stint working as a waiter before they are allowed to be a customer in a restaurant.

'Just talk to me as if I were a layman,' I said.

'I am,' he replied.

He asked me how long ago I'd lost the function in my leg, and – because he seemed quite concerned – I told him it was a few days ago. 'It was a fortnight,' J corrected me, and the surgeon looked slightly more concerned.

'I can't have made it worse by waiting, can I?' I asked, shaking my head to let him know the right answer.

His face didn't move a muscle in response but he said, 'The important thing is that we're getting it sorted now,' because doctors aren't allowed to say, 'Yes, obviously you've made it worse, you fucking dolt.' J glared burr holes into my skull.

In an effort to re-establish an air of professionalism, I shared my presumed treatment plan with the surgeon. 'So there'll be some pretty intensive physio then?' He looked at me like I'd suggested curing myself with bovine deworming pills or a protein shake. I could sense J scanning back through every single piece of medical advice I'd ever given him, assuming, not unreasonably, I'd got all that totally wrong too. The surgeon then talked me through the operation I'd need, so I opened the calendar app on my phone and asked when he wanted to do it. 'It can probably wait until 3 p.m.,' he said, slightly anxiously, and arranged for my transfer to the ward.

I lay in bed, not particularly reassured by the way the surgeon had swerved my question about how much of the function in my leg could come back. J, however, was convinced that I was going to die during my anaesthetic. I told him that it's vanishingly rare for anyone to die during an anaesthetic, then I remembered that my grandfather had died under one – so I locked that away in the vault and silently wondered if dying on an operating table was genetic. The consultant anaesthetist came round about twenty minutes later, managing to almost entirely anaesthetise our concerns with his air of calm competence. He asked if I had any allergies, looked in my mouth for some reason, then welcomed any questions.

'What are the chances he'll die under anaesthetic?' asked J.

'Oh, one in a hundred thousand,' replied the anaesthetist. 'At least. He's probably got more chance of dying by falling out of bed before the operation.' Good answer. 'Anything else?'

'Yes, sorry.' J again, with his trademark wide-eyed confidence. 'How do anaesthetics . . . work, exactly?'

'That's the funniest thing,' said the consultant, looking slightly sheepish. 'We've got no idea whatsoever. There used to be some theory about lipids, but that turned out to be nonsense. Still, the main thing is that they *do* work, right?'*

It turns out they definitely do work because three hours of total unconsciousness later, I was now the proud owner of a five-inch scar.† The surgery had apparently gone well and I would find out over the next couple of days of my hospital stay whether I'd get full strength back in my leg. I asked if I could keep my disc and the surgeon said no, of course not, so I asked why not, and he walked out the room without any explanation.

'You know,' said J, 'you are the *worst* patient.'

I wasn't having that. I explained to J that it was *my* disc and there was no reason I couldn't have it. If you have a fireplace removed from your house, you wouldn't expect the builders to refuse to let you keep it.

'Not that! The way you wasted so much time before having this seen to, the way you still act like you're a doctor, as if

---

* I don't mean to rubbish an entire specialty, but having no clue how your entire *raison d'être* does what it does seems to me like a minimum medium-sized failing.

† A strange sensation to have three hours of your existence totally missing. A sneak preview of being dead. 3/10 – not very memorable.

you're the authority on everything. The way getting medical attention is some huge inconvenience and that anyone who says otherwise is being hysterical.' Oof.

I guess my time as a doctor had taught me that I *do* know best – or at least, I mustn't ever show anyone a hint that I don't. My consultants expected it, my juniors expected it and, most of all, the patients expected it. A safe, capable pair of hands. Someone who never got tired, or made a mistake, or needed a minute to himself. How freeing it must be to hand over the reins, to sit opposite a doctor, put your complete trust in them and accept it's out of your hands. Once you've been the driver, it's hard to swap seats.

Still, as much as I was still lumbered with the odd medical idiosyncrasy, I wasn't a doctor any more.

'But also, taking the disc home. That's fucking weird too.'

Chapter 4

It didn't take many baby steps into the world of live comedy for me to realise it wasn't everything I had dreamed it was going to be. Audiences would alternate between staring back blankly like a jury desperate for their lunch break and glancing at their watches, willing the comedy magician to come on. Or there was the gig at the army barracks for a couple of thousand angry, horny squaddies. They had been drinking fairly unremittingly since they landed a few days earlier, following six months in the desert. My slot was straight after the stripper and the first empty beer can sailed onto the stage before I'd said a word. The first full beer can clonked down at my feet before I'd reached a single punchline and the head squaddie bundled me off stage for my own safety before I'd completed a full minute of material. In hindsight, I should have just started unbuttoning my shirt.

And that was the fun part. The majority of the job was spent driving. Whoever claimed it was better to travel than to arrive has never persuaded a Peugeot 206 to chug 300 miles up the M1 to the Punch and Throat pub in Carlisle. And then straight back again – there was no money for hotels: my £80 fee was already burned up in petrol.

I had a lot of time to think on those long trips up and down the country's tarmacked arteries. Time was something I'd always been short of as a doctor, ruled by rotas which monstertrucked over friendships and fun, appointments and engagements. In the car, as I followed 2 a.m. diversions, I'd think about who I used to be and how it defined me, about what I had left now that medicine was history and I was fracking my only other monetisable skill, my above-average sense of humour.

If I was going to make this work, there was something I really needed to do: I needed to fire my agent. Dear sweet Luke had his positives: he was funny, charming and efficient, and he always fought hard for my best interests. On the downside, he was fictional.

Luke was born of necessity. I discovered that to be taken seriously in my line of work, it was important to have an agent. Otherwise, I was the bloke hanging out in a playground without a child – there were quite serious questions about why I was there in the first place.

Unfortunately, much as I thought I needed an agent, when I started out, every agent I met disagreed with me. They told me, one by one, that I didn't yet have the right level of experience as a writer, despite the fact that my lack of an agent was the barrier to getting this experience. Enter Luke from LGM Talent. Over the time he represented me, his backstory fleshed out nicely – the occasional minibreak in the Lake District when a promoter asked how his weekend was, Christmas spent with his mum in Dorset. Michelle in accounts would occasionally make an appearance when invoices were due and I considered inventing Luke an assistant for extra gravitas, but the set-up was already confusing enough. As useful as it was for honing my world-building and characterisation skills, I was writing far more dialogue for my imaginary team than for any TV show.

This had worked well to begin with – and the 15 per cent

agency commission I was saving added up to many tens of pounds — until a business affairs manager from a production company wanted Luke to 'jump on the phone'. I shat myself in fear of my imminent exposure — making people laugh for all the wrong reasons.

Luke came up with several excuses why he was 'unable to come to the phone right now'. Initially, he was abroad and willing to thrash it out over his preferred medium of email, but they were happy to wait. Then Luke had a bout of laryngitis. They waited. A third excuse (A major stroke? Tongue surgery? Attacked by a wolf in the middle of Costa?) felt like one too many, so I bought a burner phone, like in *The Wire*, and begged J to pretend to be an agent called Luke. After only a few days of constant attritional nagging, J eventually agreed, on the condition that he would never have to do this for me ever again. This was for the best, really; I didn't feel J inhabited the character of Luke particularly well. He went far too thick with the Scottish accent — Luke went to Gordonstoun for fuck's sake — and portrayed a hesitancy I wouldn't expect from an agent of Luke's calibre.

After handing Luke his notice, I spent months contacting agent after agent after agent, presenting them with the random scraps of writing on my CV that they'd requested the year before. This time, the reasons for turning me down were different: their books were full; I wasn't quite the right fit for them. But eventually, someone said yes.

Normally getting an agent is a big deal for a writer — the sort of thing you'd announce to the world with a social media post that starts 'Personal news' and a klaxon emoji.* Unfortunately,

---

★ Even though it's actually 'work news'. A good agent would catch that.

everyone in my world already thought I had an agent and a lot of them had received (extremely well-written) emails from him. When I told people, 'I've got a new agent,' it implied something had gone wrong with the previous one and they'd look at me sympathetically, as if I'd said 'I've got a new kidney.'

A major perk of my newly be-agented status was that I could forward anything work-related straight on to her, because I was now far too grand to be replying to my own emails. Besides, I needed to free up my days for the ceaseless writing that was clearly just round the corner. Very usefully, it meant I could forward her the occasional email from some weird cunt with the message: 'Can you reply to this weird cunt?'

The wheels fall off this method slightly, however, if you accidentally hit 'reply' instead of 'forward'. As soon as I realised what I'd done I screamed so loudly that J ran in, assuming I'd either been electrocuted or had happened upon a picture of a first-degree relative on a specialist website. When breathlessly informed of the actual reason for my outburst, astonishingly, he came up with a workable solution: simply reply to the initial email again with something entirely innocuous, like 'I'll get back to you next week. Cheers!' and then proceed to send that same email another couple of hundred times. The weird cunt in question would obviously assume that I'd fallen foul of some outbox-based technical glitch and would open one, maybe two messages before spotting the gremlin in the works and deleting the whole lot. Unable to come up with a better plan, I pressed send. Again and again and again.

Ugh. This wouldn't have happened with Luke. But still, I had a real, human, agent – I'd stepped with both feet into life 2.0 – that deal with Paramount Pictures for a trilogy of film scripts and five comedy specials was surely just days away.

On the phone with my mum for our fortnightly catch-up, I told her my news. 'I've got a new . . .' She interrupted me, hopefully. 'Stethoscope?'*

---

* I recounted my email catastrophe to my friend Emily the same evening at drinks and she was able to spectacularly one-up me. One morning, while mindlessly leafing through Facebook, she spotted that her ex had a new girlfriend and so, as is irresistible, she launched into a full forensic investigation, clicking through a recent holiday photo album, one picture at a time, with increasing indignation. The two of them on the plane. Pfft, economy class – should have stuck with me, pal. Click. The loved-up pair in their hotel room. Pfft, did you have to pay extra for that stunning view of the carpark? The breakfast buffet. OK, fine, that does look delicious. Click. Hand in hand at the gates of Universal Studios, with more filters than the Kenco factory. Dramatic eye-roll – there's no filter for tacky though, is there? Click. The pair of them either side of a huge statue of Homer Simpson, each of them kissing his cheek, both clearly pretending to find this more fun than it actually is. Click. And then came the gut-churning lurch of the soul normally associated with dropping your only set of car keys into the Mariana Trench. Emily noticed that she had somehow managed to tag herself in that photo. As Homer. Frankly, I found it extraordinary that she was out at these drinks; I'd be living off-grid in the suburbs of Nicaragua if that had happened to me.

– FLASHBACK –

Above-Average Sense Of Humour

I'd spent the first eighteen years of my life, at the expense of almost everything else, preparing to one day become a doctor. The messaging started subliminally, as a toddler who played with syringes in the bath and learned his fine motor coordination by stacking specimen pots. Daddy day-care took place, pre-GDPR, in the smoky patient records room of his surgery. Our house was littered with medical journals, their disgusting front covers desensitising me to pictures of gangrenous genitalia and guinea worm disease. And it was impossible not to be fascinated by the antique medical ephemera on the shelves, from bone saws to tonsil guillotines.*

When secondary school came around, I became a wide-eyed, wide-beaked gosling, force-fed the corn that would eventually lead to its starring role in a foie gras starter. My evenings, weekends and holidays were stuffed with exam revision, interview practice, work experience and

---

* Had a spot of tonsillitis in the 1880s? Your doctor would tell you to open wide, then hook the guillotine around your tonsil and squeeze the handle. In one move, a blade would slice the tonsil clean off and a trident prong would snare it. Tonsil guillotines fell out of fashion because they caused a bit too much bleeding to death.

med-school-mandated extra-curricular activities. There definitely wasn't any time spare for socialising. When I left school, I was able to count my close friends on the fingers of one Twix. Still, it had paid off. All that hard work had got me into medical school.

It might have been the family trade but, like the brothel-keeper's daughter, I was in the dark about what it actually involved. All I knew was that my dad worked *a lot*. He'd drop us off at school on his way to surgery, a full hour and a half before assembly, so we'd sit in the computer 'lab' and play solitaire until all the part-timers arrived. In the evening, he wouldn't get home until long after dinner. Whenever I tried to discover what was keeping him out of the house for fourteen hours a day, I never got much of an answer, like if you asked, 'How was your day?' to a contract killer or a philanderer. He'd generally bat away my questions with a stack of silly or disgusting anecdotes, a showreel of harmless diversions that never got close enough to the truth that I might be put off. 'Did I tell you about the home visit where the man hoarded hardcore pornography? It was like a warehouse – there must have been 50,000 magazines!'

And finally my dream was fulfilled. Well, someone's dream, but . . . whatever. Now wasn't the time to pick nits, now was the time to reinvent myself – a life full of friends, parties and laughter awaited.

Unfortunately, catching up on eighteen years of social skills was trickier than I'd imagined. I'd been coddled and constricted by single-sex education to the point of preposterousness, with the first quarter of my life expectancy spent barely speaking to a human female (leading to, among other things, my use of the phrase 'human female'). Elton John was wrong about sorry being the hardest word

– for me, it was 'hello'. I would walk across to a table full of other medic freshers at lunchtime, or down to a busy row in the lecture theatre, practising an insouciant 'mind if I join you?' in my head, before awkwardness and fear of rejection took hold of my confidence and squashed it like a moth. I'd sit elsewhere and promise myself I'd try again the next day. And the next day. And the next day.

Sometimes, the loneliest feelings of all don't come from total isolation but from being on the edge of the crowd, watching the rest of the world live its life, as if it's happening on television and not three feet away from you in the canteen. But I told myself that maybe this was just what adulthood was like sometimes.

One day, a few months into my first year, having made very little progress beyond thanking people for holding open doors, I was sitting at a table on my own, a vision in Topman, eating my omelette baguette* in the med school building, when someone sat down next to me.

'Hi, I'm Mike.'

Fuck. Oh god. Say something normal, Adam. I looked up. Happily it wasn't an eighteen-year-old Mike but a middle-aged Jewish Mike, and after a lifetime of being paraded out in front of my parents' friends to play the piano or recite some Pliny at their dinner parties, I knew how to speak to these ones.

---

* Your 'normal' is simply what you're exposed to until you know different. At school, the canteen was called the 'buttery', the medical room the 'sanitarium' and the school shop the 'commissariat'. It took time for me to realise that these were weird, made-up names that had to be excised from my vocabulary. Similarly at university, the café we all used specialised in cheese and onion omelette baguettes and like everything else, we just accepted it. Who knew it was pizza-on-toast levels of weird?

'You like your own company, then?' he asked. He had a kind face. People always say that, usually when they're trying to think of a more diplomatic way of saying someone isn't attractive. But it wasn't that. He just had a kind face. I knew I'd be able to reply honestly with no fear of judgement.

'Not especially.'

He'd spotted me sitting on my own a few times, he said. He was a pharmacology lecturer. He wanted to check everything was OK with me. He took an interest in his students' welfare. An interest in my welfare – this was new.

Mike Schachter spoke in a lilting mid-European accent, his speech peppered with well-constructed witticisms and bons mots. It felt like I was in a film, and this kindly Hungarian man had joined me on a park bench and was offering the excellent advice I would need if I was to make it unscathed into the second act.

'Medicine is a job where you need friends,' he told me, 'because the job won't always be your friend.' When I confessed I was struggling a little in that department, he said I just needed to find my tribe.

What were my interests? Did I play hockey or table tennis or the cello? I shrugged. I'd told my parents I'd joined the orchestra, but I hadn't. Nor did I intend to. As much as I used to love playing music, doing it as a calculated move to get into medical school had sort of killed it for me. Mike wasn't deterred. Might I enjoy the orthopaedic surgery society,* he wondered, or a little light opera? What about Médecins Sans Frontières? Rock climbing? I hoped

---

* What would a group of banging and nailing enthusiasts even get up to? Day trips to B&Q?

my lack of interest wasn't coming across as ingratitude. How about writing sketches for the Soirée – the medical school's age-old end-of-year revue, where students make fun of conditions, consultants and professors? He must have spotted a glint of something in my eye because he scribbled down my details and promised to introduce me to Agatha, who ran the Soirée. 'We'll find you your tribe.'

People talk a lot about medics' dark sense of humour but maybe don't realise how much it's actively cultivated.* These end-of-year revues are financed and readily encouraged by medical schools, and are attended by the majority of students, who lap them up, regardless of quality. Whether it's as an outlet for emotion, to release tension or to bond people together in difficult situations, gallows humour is found in all extreme environments – medicine, the military, firefighters, the police. Even in concentration camps.† It's a form of resistance, and it's the only coping mechanism that doctors are usually ever taught.

Mike would check in on me every few weeks but was never intrusive. I appreciated his influence. Just knowing there was someone looking out for me, even in the deep background, helped me finally start to nose my way out of my shell. The act of writing itself also helped. Putting words on a page – whatever they are – means there are fewer of them jangling around inside your head. I was

---

* Former doctors made up 17 per cent of Monty Python, 33 per cent of The Goodies and 100 per cent of Harry Hill.

† As the doctor and philosopher Viktor Frankl says in his Auschwitz memoir, *Man's Search for Meaning,* 'Humour, more than anything else in the human make-up, can afford an aloofness and an ability to rise above any situation, even if only for a few seconds.'

terrible. The sketches I wrote would have silenced a pack of hysterical hyenas. But then I'd have been useless at rock climbing and badminton too. It didn't really matter. I was meeting people and having fun.

I made friends slowly but surely, and certainly more easily when I eventually discovered that everyone, to some degree or other, was either scared or pretending not to be. Ultimately, the whole world is winging it. It's just that some people are better at hiding it – doctors especially.

By the time we got to the night of the Soirée itself, I wasn't quite reborn, but I certainly felt different to the buttoned-up mouse I'd been just a few months earlier. I had a lot more to say for myself and a lot more to offer. Mike came to watch that year's performance and sent me a card of congratulations after the show. Really it should have been me sending him a card.

In my second year, Mike wasn't in touch so much, he could see I was integrating into medical school life; his work was done and he was probably off nurturing another nest of mice. Meanwhile, I was now one of the Soirée 'officers', with responsibility for putting together that year's production. Top of the to-do list was deciding on the show's name – traditionally a medical pun based on a famous film title. Think *28 Days Late, Good Will Huntington's* or *The Importance of Seeing Hernias*. At our third meeting, I came up with what I thought was the perfect title, seamlessly melding a current Matt Damon blockbuster with the biggest medical story of the century: *The Talented Dr Shipman.*

The ink was barely dry on the posters before I was summoned to the Dean's office to explain myself. A year earlier, I imagine I'd have been too meek to argue my case, but the new, more self-assured me took no time to launch into a vigorous defence of my tasteless pun. I repeated what I'd been told by his own staff about medicine's 'necessary tradition of dark humour'. The Dean insisted that the title was 'unacceptable' and that it was 'bringing the medical school into disrepute'.

He was right, of course. There's a line, which I had crossed in my desire for a cheap laugh. I apologised and I meant it. He thanked me for my apology and said he would bear it in mind. The only question he had was whether to suspend me or expel me. Apparently it really was that serious. I would receive a letter in due course. Shit.

The idea of it all crashing to a bitter end because of a bad joke was more than I could bear, so I went and sat in Mike's office and I begged him to help. I wasn't entirely sure why – by now I wasn't 100 per cent convinced I wanted to be a doctor any more. But what else was I going to do? Added to which, I felt I'd only just begun to find myself, *like* myself even. I was having fun. Finally! Good clean fun with human males and females who had become friends. I really didn't want it to end.

Mike told me to leave it with him and, presumably thanks to his intervention, the anticipated punishment from the Dean never did turn up in my pigeonhole. Instead there was one short, scrawled note from Mike: a little joke, I think. 'Maybe we need to find you a different tribe.'*

---

* To think I could have avoided all this by going with *Star Wards Episode I: The Phantom Meningitis*.

Chapter 5

Much as I wanted to forget my time on labour ward, it was all but impossible to avoid, like having a tinsel allergy in December. Leaving the job didn't stop friends from treating me as a permanent on-call helpline for anything remotely pregnancy or infertility related. And not even inner-circle friends (if you can call one person a circle), but anyone who ever knew I was an obstetrician: the girl who lived next to me in university halls and I never got round to unfriending on Facebook and – trauma squared! – the estate agent who had sold on my marital home. Another reminder arrived in an A4 manila envelope, the kind that almost always brings bad news.

Dear Dr Kay,
Thank you for your interest in Medacs. Please find enclosed
registration documents for the role of OBSTETRIC
REGISTRAR. Please indicate if you are looking for a
LOCUM or PERMANENT role, and which geographical
regions would suit.

I hadn't expressed any interest whatsoever in working as a locum, but someone clearly had. Someone who had my postal address. I was about to phone my mother – it might as well have had her lipstick on the stamp – when I realised I couldn't be bothered with the fight. And it wasn't *necessarily* her.

It hadn't entirely escaped J's attention that he'd been paying for every single bill, round of drinks and supermarket trip. His tentative enquiries as to whether it might make sense for me to find a day job – just a little stopgap, something to tide us over, how about the odd shift in a shop, maybe? – were met with fury. Overnight success takes years! Would Shakespeare have written *King Lear* if he'd spent ten hours a day stacking instant noodles at Budgens? Fuck that shit.

But god works in mysterious ways for someone who doesn't exist, and sent me salvation a few days later in the form of the biggest opportunity of my life by a factor of twenty: to adapt a Broadway musical for the West End. It would involve working for a company whose name I probably wouldn't have mentioned anyway, even without the Mickey Mouse non-disclosure agreement they made me sign. Let's call them Bisney. The brief was to go through the script of this musical line by line and make it UK-friendly. Anything peculiar to America – any jokes or cultural references that might puzzle a UK audience, any linguistic quirks or unacceptably poor grammar – were to be weeded out and replaced with a cavalcade of proper English gorblimey zingers.* Might I be interested, they wondered.

I said yes, keeping my cool as much as I could, which wasn't very much. A few days later, they wondered if I'd be able to fly over to New York for a week to watch the original show

---

* Step one: converting sidewalks to pavements and trunks to boots must always be performed manually. The UK edition of *The Great Leader and the Fighter Pilot* by Blaine Harden was the victim of an automated find-and-replace job, and so includes the word 'particitrousers'.

and really get to know it. You know what? I reckoned I could probably make that work.

This was it, the Big Bang of my writing career. Suddenly, my career path no longer resembled a helicopter whose rotor had stopped mid-flight. My name might not yet be up in lights, but at least the lights back home might stay on. The best part about getting good news is telling people – friends, family, teachers who said you'd never amount to anything, the guy who works the lottery machine at Chiswick Sainsbury's. I told J, who was genuinely delighted and could see this being the accelerant my career needed. I told my mum, who replied that heavy rain was forecast for the next few days, which meant that her Nordic walking was probably off.

I'm sure oligarchs get tired of opulent hotel rooms with gold trim but I vowed never to forget the feeling as I stepped nervously into my five-star hotel room, an Executive Deluxe, no less. My itinerary was waiting for me there and involved . . . oh. Watching the show eight times over the course of the week – every single matinee and evening performance. Bisney weren't fucking around; they wanted me to really, *really* get to know this show. Which of course I was happy to do. Mostly because there was no choice: I had to retrieve the tickets from the box office at every performance, so they'd find out if I bunked off.

First show. I collected my ticket and two drinks tokens, one of which I swapped for a Diet Coke, then went to the fourth row of the stalls to watch the show. It was fun, although I'm not sure it added anything to my knowledge of the script, which had already been amply satisfied by reading it.

Second show. Same procedure. I procured myself a Diet Coke and took it to the fourth row of the stalls. At the interval, I decided I'd earned a proper drink, so I had a glass of borderline-acceptable Sauvignon Blanc.

Third show. I went straight for the wine and the lady at the bar suggested I trade my token for the whole bottle, rather than just a glass. 'It's valid for anything we serve, Sir.' Fucking hell – this was a game-changer. I took her up on this kind offer. At the interval, I ordered a second bottle of plonk and the rest of the show simply rocketed by. I felt like I'd found the cheat mode on this slightly repetitive game.

Fourth show. I was mouthing along with every syllable. It was a form of Walter torture. I was pretty sure I could understudy for every single member of the cast. Well, in the first half at least. I'm not sure what my footwork would be like after my interval drink.

Eighth show. No recall of the previous three – I imagine they were exactly the same as the preceding ten thousand the cast had performed. By now, I was kicking off with four shots of vodka topped up with Diet Coke in a special reusable branded cup the size of a kitchen bin, and then seeing in the second half with a bottle of prosecco. It wasn't just that the show was now mind-numbing, there was also a creeping feeling of depression that my career break wasn't quite what I'd begged the universe for. When you wish upon a star, my anus. Still, if I'd learned one thing at medical school it's that you can get through pretty much anything if you have a glass of wine or six. And in this job, I didn't even have to wait until I got home.

Back in Blighty, I spent the next fortnight working solidly on the script. I put in shifts: twelve hours flat out – writing, editing, fine-tuning and finessing. Ignoring the clock and J's calls to come to bed or have a sandwich or 'have a shower, it's been three days'. This is something I knew how to do, from the days when lives depended on it. And then I'd reward myself with a week's worth of alcohol units in an hour. Something else I knew how to do.

I delivered a 50-page document fizzing with Brit-tastic jokes and references, offering multiple alternatives wherever there was the slightest whiff of a star or a stripe. The producer thanked me for my hard work and it only took a month for the showtunes in my head to fade, like a gay version of tinnitus. It had been worth it, though. I was happy with the work I'd done. And after all, if I impressed Bisney, who knew what might come next . . .

A few months later, the show was set to open in the West End and Bisney had posted me a pair of tickets. Having only recently recovered from my immersion in it, my instinct was to hide them, but J seemed very excited to hear the results of my first crack at writing for an audience of more than about ten people, so we went along.

In the foyer afterwards, J was extremely positive. He'd enjoyed it, he said, and had laughed a lot. He had. I'd heard him. A switch had been flicked, I could tell – he was finally on board, pumped for where this could take my career. I should probably get my agent to check in with Bisney in a couple of weeks, he said, strike while the iron is hot, while my name was still in their heads and the newsprint fresh on the inevitable rapturous reviews. Who knows what other projects they've got coming up, he said – maybe we should stay for a drink and see if I could 'bump into anyone'? I said I was tired and would rather get home.

When we got back, J asked me how many of my jokes they'd used. I said I hadn't been counting, which wasn't quite true. I had been counting and the total was zero. I poured myself a pint of wine and dug out that letter from the locum agency – you know, just in case.

– FLASHBACK –

A Glass Of Wine Or Six

Chest compressions, we were taught at medical school, are performed at the speed of *The Archers'* theme tune.* Rumpy pumpy pumpy pum, Rumpy pumpy pah pah. How could I ever forget that? We would stand round tables in class and practise on amputated plastic torsos, which gave a reassuring click when you pressed their sternum deep enough, humming along to *The Archers*, giving the room a certain 'lunchtime at the old people's home' ambience.

And then, six months later, on an A&E placement, I saw CPR being performed in earnest for the first time. Pietro, one of the SHOs, ushered a couple of us into a cubicle for a ringside view. A woman in her sixties or seventies was splayed on a bed. I didn't know whether her heart had stopped when she was in the department or if she was brought in that way. In fact, I didn't know anything about her, beyond the fact her heart had stopped and a small crowd of people were trying to restart it.

---

* For readers outside of BBC Radio 4's broadcast area, the Bee Gees' *Stayin' Alive* also works very well, pleasingly.

A nurse was pushing hard down onto her naked chest – grunting through the effort, his sweat dripping onto her unperfused skin, spittle flying as he counted his compressions. Nobody was humming the theme tune to anything. The cubicle smelled overpoweringly of urine – whether hers or a previous occupant's. The lights were bright and oppressive; I felt like I was intruding on a private moment.

Her chest wall was bending beyond the rules of physics – perhaps her ribs were snapping; I wouldn't have been able to hear above the A&E kerfuffle. Her eyes were rolled back into her head, her mouth was slack, her lips greyed out and thin. An arm jolted with every compression, its hand flopping in response. I saw a wedding ring, eroded by years of rubbing for good luck or taking on and off to do the washing up. A life was both materialising and draining away right before my eyes.

I don't know how her story ended. I looked at my watch and said to no one in particular that I needed to go to a tutorial, even though no one cared and no one was listening, then slipped out through the curtain, quick-walked across the department and ran outside to gulp some cold Ealing air. I'm not sure what I felt more sick about – the brutal indignity of CPR or the fact I couldn't even watch it. Great doctor I'll be!

But it was a Friday and that meant there was a Bop at the med school bar. Bops, hops, sports' nights, balls: whatever day of the week it was, there was always a spurious excuse to take refuge in vast amounts of university-subsidised alcohol. Which is how I found myself participating in a ritual* called The Centurion.

The rules of The Centurion are very simple: you drink a shot of beer, then one minute later, you drink another shot of beer, then you repeat this for one hundred minutes and one hundred shots of beer. One final rule – you're not allowed to leave the bar till it's over. Most of the drinking games I took part in, as a rather desperate way to try to fit in, involved things like bedpans full of gin and eventually collapsing unconscious outside the hospital the bar was inexplicably housed in. The Centurion was an outlier in that it didn't get you incapably drunk. I mean, you wouldn't want to be in command of a passenger jet after playing but it's still 'only' four pints of beer in an hour and a half. It challenges your body in a different way: how long can your bladder hold three times more liquid than it was designed to? You'd better hope the answer is one hundred minutes.

---

* The most dangerous bar game bar none in medical school folklore is the Sux Race. It's hopefully apocryphal but knowing medical students as I do, I can just about believe it existed. The rules are simple: participants line up at the starting post and on the referee's whistle, they're injected in the leg with a syringeful of suxamethonium – and they're off! As fast as they can, for as long as they can. Usually found on the anaesthetics trolley, suxamethonium is not exactly what you might call a party drug. Neither is it performance-enhancing, as it paralyses all of the muscles in your body. Great if you're having your appendix out, rather less useful if you're racing round a sticky student bar. You collapse after seconds, and the person whose body falls furthest from the starting line is the winner.

Unfortunately, suxamethonium doesn't discriminate between the muscles required for running and those required for breathing. If your peers are unable to perform some competent bag-valve-mask ventilation – which, due to their levels of drunkenness and incompetence, is highly likely – then you're dead. But on the plus side, it might make a great anecdote eighty years later for a researcher on *Who Do You Think You Are?*

As you drink and try to Paul McKenna your urinary tract into complying, you're serenaded by a chorus of 'rugby songs'. The one that still haunts me slates students of a rival medical school, shouting out that they're 'high-born fairies'. Not the easiest chant to get behind when you have fairy tendencies yourself.

My poor bladder fought valiantly but around twenty shots from the end, my body found itself unable to house a piss-filled zeppelin. Protocol dictated that, rather than go running to the loo like a poof (their words), I should remain seated at the bar and soak my jeans. And so I did, to huge cheers.*

The Centurion might have done its job. I would have forgotten all about my day in A&E if the stench of urine didn't bring me straight back into that cubicle. Another drink?

---

* Considered among the pantheon of medical school greats is the fuckwit who, after completing The Centurion, went on to spend the night in an operating theatre with a torn bladder and urine sloshing around his abdomen, causing life-threatening peritonitis. Two nights in ITU! Legend!

Chapter 6

J suggested joining me for our family Christmas on the basis that we'd been dating for almost two years. I counterbid with doing it in twenty years' time, in the hope that we'd compromise somewhere around the ten year mark, but he wasn't in the haggling mood. My mother wasn't making it easy either. 'It's unfair on your grandmother if she turns up and he's just *here*,' she explained. 'You need to warn her in advance.' Warn her. Do people need 'warning' that there might be gay people in any room they're about to enter?

I said I would just handle it on the day – perhaps we could wear matching 'HO-HO-HOMO' Christmas jumpers? My mother said that if I was going to be like that, J couldn't come at all. (Fine by me!) I asked why she couldn't simply mention the fact that I'm gay at some point in the build-up to Christmas – think of it as a kind of advent treat! – and she said that she wasn't doing my dirty work for me. Warnings, dirty work – I didn't need to fetch the illustrated dictionary from my childhood bedroom to understand what this conversation was really about.

We almost launched into a full-blown argument, until I realised that, in actual fact, she was probably the last person on earth I'd want breaking the news; it would be like having General Pinochet officiate your wedding.

To be fair, we have a complicated history on this topic. When I first came out to my parents at university, they provided the standard briefing that it was just a phase and I hadn't found the right girl yet.★ They must have felt vindicated in their opinion when, a bunch of years later, I married H. I can say that I married her with the best intentions and for the right reasons, even if they don't look great on paper now. In my mind, it wasn't a case of hiding who I really was, rather celebrating that I had finally become the person society wanted me to be. I had fallen in love with a wonderful woman who loved me back and we were launching into an exciting future together. How could it possibly be a deception when we both wanted the same thing? It was day one of the rest of my life: a new beginning, a new me.

But of course the feelings didn't fade – they never do. Their intensity waxed and waned but they didn't go anywhere – a background hum that no amount of jamming cotton buds in my ears would ever drown out. I loved her, but clearly not in the way I needed to. In those first few weeks after the truth became unavoidable, I was broken. I left medicine and ended my marriage within a matter of months – it wasn't so much ripping off a plaster as bursting out of the barbed wire wound tightly around me. It's a sad fact that the path to one's own

---

★ Long before we met, J struggled for many months to come to terms with the realisation that he was gay and was particularly tortured by the thought of telling his family. He was so keen to avoid having 'the conversation' that he would take to his bed for weeks on end. Reasoning that he was depressed and not really sure what else to do about it, his family took every opportunity to rally his spirits with upbeat stories and good news. As he sat hunched miserably over his cornflakes one morning, his Catholic grandmother excitedly rustled her newspaper at him. 'This will cheer you up!' she exclaimed. J girded himself. What would it be? Had 5ive reformed? No. 'The Pope has said that gay marriage is an abomination!'

happiness is often paved with the heartbreak of others – or maybe that's just what every selfish person tells themselves. The guilt, many years in the making, took a long time to subside – and it's still there, plain to see under karmic blacklight.

In the end, I decided to collect my grandmother early on Christmas morning and while driving I would explain to her about the bees and the bees. As I pootled over to her house, I spent the entire time rehearsing the exact phrasing I would use. And then I spent half an hour sat outside her driveway debating whether to tell her at all. She could always just meet J while I went to the bathroom or faked my own death.

It wasn't like she'd expressed particularly old-fashioned views in the past – a wealth of age and experience might even have expanded her worldview? Unlike some other members of my family, she hadn't cared about me quitting the day job, so why would she care about this? But then again, she was a woman in her late eighties, so the odds were always loaded towards the opposite response. You never quite know how someone's going to react when you come out. The first time might be *the big one*, when you first say the words. But the truth is, you actually come out every few days, for the rest of your life. To the hotel receptionist who wants to confirm that it's definitely a double bed you require, not a Bert-and-Ernie twin arrangement.★ To the mortgage advisor who assumes that J and I are colleagues. To the odious Max Clifford who, thanks to J's job, we found ourselves opposite at some charity dinner and asked us, 'What's

---

★ I once wrote to a hotel manager after one such incident, explaining in the politest terms (of which I'm capable) that assuming two men aren't a couple and questioning them on it is a latent form of societal homophobia and one that could perhaps be handled more sensitively. The reply came back 'Dear Dr and Mrs Kay'.

the deal with you two?' and then flopped his wrist forward theatrically with a Kenneth Williams 'Oooooooh!' when we told him.* They might make their excuses, turn away and talk to someone else. There might just be a slight dip in their gaze,† as if continuing to lock eyes with you will result in them contracting homosexuality. Perhaps their face will change entirely and they'll reach into the cellar that once contained their soul and haul out some of their favourite slurs. They might even offer you a physical manifestation of their disapproval – although I've personally never been thumped for it, for which I accept I'm both lucky and begrudgingly grateful.

My hesitancy wasn't just about my congenital inability to open up. I guess it was largely because my grandmother had never had to entertain the possibility that I had a sex life before: our relationship had always been so innocent, and suddenly I was inviting her to picture me fucking a bloke.‡ Ugh, right. Time to do this. I knocked on her front door then helped her into the car.

As we drove, I decided that it wasn't quite the time to do this. Maybe I'd have a bit of a catch-up with her first – just for ten minutes. Twenty minutes. An hour and a half. We were five minutes from my parents' house when I finally grabbed the bull by the balls.

---

* It was especially galling that Max Clifford disapproved of homosexuality, given it later transpired that he was keen to have sex with almost anyone, regardless of such trifles as consent or adulthood.

† Pun partially intended.

‡ I always reckon that's what goes through someone's mind when you come out to them – it's why homophobes can't deal with the concept of gay people. They could just about cope with a couple of lads being close friends, going to the opera, maybe even holding hands at a push, but only if they have Ken-Doll-style genitalia-free groins.

I said the first part really casually, as rehearsed. 'I just wanted to say that I've met someone new, and we're living together'.

'Oh, that's lovely!' replied Grandma.

Then, at a much faster pace, as if I was reading the T&Cs for a payday loan: 'He's called J, by the way, and he's going to be joining us for Christmas dinner, so you'll meet him today.'

At this point her face fell and she stared at the road ahead in absolute silence. 'Oh no, Adam,' she tutted. 'Oh dear.' My heart sank. The spectre of a ruined Christmas turned in my stomach. Then she added, almost forcing me to pull over on the hard shoulder of the M26 and give her a hug, 'I haven't bought him a present.'

– FLASHBACK –

The Big One

Today, it's fair to say that pornography is as common as the muck it is. In 1993, when I started secondary school and before the internet had democratised smut, it was a very different kettle of filth. Beyond the odd torn-out *Razzle* centrefold left in the bushes by visiting perverts, curious teenage minds and hands had little to work with other than their imaginations and the Vaseline in the bathroom cabinet.

Sam Wilson was the only person in my class who had access to the internet and, by extension, access to porn. I presume that the *Guinness Book of Records* doesn't have a category for 'Youngest Porn Baron' but Sam's entrepreneurial spirit would have made him a firm contender. He would trawl bulletin boards from the proto-version of the web on his family computer, then print out reams of erotica.

Sam stuffed his locker with lever-arch files, each subdivided into different categories containing dozens of plastic wallets full of printouts. Sam's contraband was quite quaint in retrospect: no pneumatic models or grainy money shots, just hardcore pornographic essays. Page after page of pistoning, squelching X-rated Mills and Boon. This Mini-Hefner ran a louche lending library, letting each document go out overnight for 50p, or £1 at the weekend. It took me a few weeks after hearing about his enterprise to pluck up the courage to make a withdrawal. When I finally sidled up to him, he opened his locker, pulled out the smut, looked me up and down and said, like a shoemaker sizing my feet, 'You're gay, right?'

At that point I had never entertained such a consideration. My life thus far had been a sexless blur of algebra homework and piano practice, with precious little else in between. But now he came to mention it, there had been something a little off that I hadn't been able to put my finger on. I felt something of an outsider in the usual playground discussions about which girls we all fancied, as if my personal radio wasn't tuned to the same station as everyone else's. I guess it would explain why I enjoyed being rugby tackled slightly more than I should, a particular interest in *Blue Peter* whenever Tim Vincent did a swimming challenge, and that decidedly feverous dream about Clint Barton in 5R1 . . . the way his hair fell over his eyes made me feel like I'd just got off a roundabout. But now something I had never really thought about beyond 'Oh that's a bit weird, never mind, back to the saxophone' needed to be addressed quite urgently.

It's difficult to know how to answer a direct 'Are you gay?' at the best of times – people are usually asking because they want to fuck you or fuck you up – but even as a schoolkid who'd never been asked it before, it felt like a trap. School was an environment where any vague divergence from the norm was pointed out loudly and with shrieks of disgust; I didn't want to be Rick Jones, who could bend his arms round his back and stick his fingers in opposite nostrils, or Carl Burbank with his webbed penis. Why would I choose to invite difference, bullying, ridicule? More importantly, what did this mean for the path laid clearly out for me: a doctor with a nice life and a nice house, a nice wife and a couple of well-behaved children?

But . . . he wasn't wrong. He'd read me like the *Great Gatsby* in my satchel. Did everyone else know too? Was it in the way I spoke, moved, breathed, held my pen? As pivotal as the moment clearly was, I had the more urgent dilemma of not wanting to waste a hard-earned quid on porn that wasn't going to make me hit the high note.

'Yeah, I think so.'

He rifled through a file to find the right section. I felt sick with bender's remorse. 'You . . . won't tell anyone, right?'

Sam shrugged. He was the custodian of a whole year-group's sexual secrets – the dark web of 1993 – the only thing he cared about was the cold hard currency of cash so he could buy death metal CDs and clear the tuck shop of Chewits. So I parted with my pound and that weekend, thanks to Sam Wilson, and the story of an Australian pick-up truck driver,* I came out to myself. Again and again and again. I still get a reflex erection whenever I see a Toyota Hilux.†

---

* The driver picked up a hitchhiker in the outback and, in a rather forward move, suggested that he should penetrate the hitchhiker using a banana as a makeshift dildo. Despite the fact that one might expect a banana in such heat wouldn't have the requisite rigidity, this was nonetheless a resounding success, with ejaculations all round. The third act of the story was that the driver then ate it. (The banana, not the hitchhiker.)

† Or a banana.

Chapter 7

Despite tying you into the commitment of a mortgage for thirty years, owning your own place feels like freedom. It's somewhere to store your crap without the threat of a landlord 'just popping in' to make sure you haven't taken the plastic covers off the sofa, that you can decorate or furnish as you want, instead of spending your life inside whichever home interiors trend your landlord saw on *DIY SOS* in 2004.

After I left medicine, it felt important to get back onto the property ladder, albeit on a lower rung. It would mean that I hadn't checked out of the real world completely, that giving up my job hadn't been a huge mistake. That I wasn't just floating round untethered, but I had a firm mooring in life. Plus ideally, I'd be able to live somewhere with more square feet than decibels.

So I saved. Like a demon. If it wasn't keeping me alive or covering a non-negotiable bill, every single centime I earned was spirited away into my dusty savings account. Saving also meant doing things I wouldn't normally do for money. While I managed to avoid the oldest profession – I'm not sure my self-esteem could have handled finding out the street value of my penis – I did the writerly equivalent: composing wedding speeches for swaggering City boys. They might have known about investment banking and sexually harassing their female colleagues but they knew fuck all about stringing a sentence together. What they wanted was a set of standard, horrific, best man or groom jokes personalised in words short enough for their coke-fuddled brains to get around.★ My soul eroded away but I kept my eyes on the mooring.

And yet it wasn't enough. Me and the mortgage company had very different ideas about what this mooring might look like – it would be a lot smaller than I'd hoped and the zone number would be a lot higher.†

Thankfully, Zoopla allows you to sort every property in London by lowest price. Page one – where I'd be picking from – was the domain of the derelict garage with a fan heater that had somehow found its way into the wrong search results or the almost-as-unappealing studio flat: houses chunked up by (presumably evil) property developers into separate lockable cells.

Five months later, we had spent 100 per cent of our worldly worth on a property slightly larger than a Fiat Brava. Number 17b had neither kerb appeal, the 'X factor', charm, potential or anything else that TV property shows had conditioned me to look for, and it was comically worse than the place I'd had as a doctor a few years earlier. But by pooling our resources, we had achieved what for many people is only a dream – a place that was all ours. Well, 5 per cent of it was; the other 95 per cent belonged to the red-jacketed shysters at Santander.

The concept of a studio flat is quite well-established: pretty

---

★ I'm so nervous that this is the fifth time today I've stood up from a warm seat with a piece of paper in my hand. I'll be quick – I want to jump on my wife like a wolf on a panini. Copy, paste. Copy, paste.

† My income was in fact described as 'derisory' (Santander, 2013).

much everything is in one room – kitchen, bedroom and living area. 17b took this concept to its logical conclusion, and included the bathroom within the 'all in one'. To give the property developer shark one nineteenth of a percentage point of credit, they did at least attempt to segregate the bathroom with some standalone half-height saloon doors, which provided modesty from the occasional angle. As the bathroom had no sink, we'd brush our teeth in the kitchen and spit on the crockery like some kind of tattooed hustler in a C movie. I could convince myself I'd done the right thing with my life, just as long as I closed my eyes. Plus ears and nose, if J was taking a shit while I was watching *Newsnight*.

We decided that we could probably improve on the shitting set-up: a bit of reconfiguration and the odd extra wall could turn our un-des-res into a bona fide one-bedroom flat. And after a second year of forsaking takeaways, evenings out and anything else vaguely approaching fun, we'd saved enough cash to fix it up.

All we needed to do now was hire our architect and project manager, followed by a builder, then recruit the key trades of plumber, electrician, plasterer and decorator. Because our savings only ran to the materials we'd need for the project, I applied for – and was successful in securing – every single one of these roles. I didn't have any experience, but how hard could it be? And as J pointed out, it wasn't like I was doing much else with my days.

I sketched the flat's new layout freehand on graph paper that I bought specially on a 3-for-2 from Smith's, then spent countless days cruising kitchen showrooms, DIY stores and bathroom suppliers choosing everything from my dream flooring (anything below £20 a square metre that wasn't plastic grass) to my dream bath (under £300 and narrow enough to fit into a space the size of a coffin). Between a rabbit hole of internet forums, YouTube videos and a solid fortnight bingeing *Grand Designs*, I did acquire some genuine superficial expertise.

J was away producing a TV show* across the two months of the 'build', as we architects say, so I was on my own 'on site', as we project managers say.

In medicine, every operation, every procedure, every task can be boiled down to a simple list of instructions. Whether you're putting in a drip or separating conjoined twins,† you start at the start and move one step at a time until you're at the end. The same applied to renovating a flat. I wasn't fast and I wasn't achieving perfection, but I was getting there. As my mum used to say about my piano playing, 'slow but inaccurate'.

Despite the savings on staff costs, I still couldn't afford to stay anywhere offsite, so I had to get slightly creative. The only part of the flat that didn't require renovation was an alcove the size of a large wardrobe adjacent to the living (/sleeping/dining/washing/shitting) area. I moved every single object, piece of furniture or keepsake that we owned into the alcove and somehow Tetris-ed it all in. I then laid our mattress on top of everything, about five feet above the ground, accessible only by climbing onto a chest of drawers. In place of an actual door, I stretched a thick sheet of blue plastic across the frame and stapled it on, to protect me and all our belongings from the endless dust. It looked like the set of a loner's attic room

---

* This is where I would explain what a TV producer does, if I knew. It seems to mostly involve saying phrases like 'development slate', 'precinct' and 'authorial voice' into a telephone.

† An operation to separate conjoined twins in Singapore holds the record for the longest surgical procedure, at 103 hours. Coincidentally, the length of time it would take to watch all eleven series of *Frasier* (the phrase 'back to back' was removed from this footnote during the 'sensitivity read').

 off

76

from a particularly gruesome 'she knew her killer' episode of CSI: West London. Every evening, I would slither through a gap in the corner of the sheeting, then Blu Tack myself back in. The next morning, I'd fold myself back out again and hermetically seal away our belongings from the endless dust. My system worked pretty well, until one day the Blu Tack failed and everything we owned became coated in a thick shroud of dust. It also meant that I could no longer sleep there without contracting ultra-emphysema, so from that moment onwards, I slept in the car.

I didn't mention to J that I was sleeping in the car, mostly because I didn't need him pointing out that a sixteen-year-old Peugeot 206 wasn't a great place for someone with a history of spinal surgery to spend the night. Not that I could guarantee a decent sleep anyway – all the goose-down bedding in the world couldn't stave off my 3 a.m. blood-drenched nightmares. (Which I also hadn't told him about.) Another legacy of my job was that I couldn't think of a single doorstep I could pitch up on with my battered carry-on: it had seen me drift away from almost every friend I'd made and my break-up had seen off the remainder. When you're working 97-hour weeks, you don't really think of what life might be like when you're not. The return on my investment into the people around me was commensurate with my initial stake: zero.

It was difficult to feel pleased with my life's trajectory as I settled under the freezing blanket in a rusting Peugeot, trying not to peg myself with the gearstick. Sure, I couldn't imagine going back to labour ward but I could always retrain as a GP? How difficult could that be? Find myself a quiet rural practice, a couple of well-behaved Airedale terriers and a thatched house called Wisteria Cottage that didn't need any major renovations.

I'd just nodded off on my second night in the car when an elderly dog-walking neighbour rapped on the window to check I was OK. Rather than get into the whole thing, I pretended I'd accidentally fallen asleep, somehow in the passenger seat. When he went back indoors, I drove a few streets away so that my secret life as a car-dweller need never come to light. A week later, the same neighbour spotted me in the car again and asked if everything was OK. At that point, my reputation as local oddball was permanently established.

I phoned J the next morning to say we should sell the flat. He was pretty baffled. We'd just spent every single penny we had on the place and the renovation had been my sole occupation and topic of conversation for what seemed like a century. 'I'm just . . . not feeling it, I guess.' He suggested that we shouldn't do anything hasty – it would be finished in a couple of weeks and he'd be back home then so we could both take a view.

Sure enough, I eventually got over my mortification and was actually pretty proud of the work I'd done. J looked around and I prepared myself for the inevitable compliments.

He sighed. 'Yeah, it's not great, is it?' Then, with such unbridled honesty it made me reconsider asking him if I looked nice in an outfit ever again, he launched into what quickly became an evisceration of everything he despised about my grand design – specifically, all of it. The colour choices, the flooring, the taps that apparently looked exactly like his nan's. The tiling was 'slapdash'; the kitchen units were 'wonkier than medieval teeth' and the bathroom floor sloped so much you could 'slalom down it'. He hated the positioning of the toilet, which was admittedly a *touch* too close to the wall, but I dispute that he had to 'shit side-saddle, like a nineteenth-century noblewoman'.

I wanted to defend my vision but how could I now force him to live in a flat he hated from grout to glazing? And so we loaded up Zoopla again and sorted every property in London from low to high.

– FLASHBACK –

A Quiet Rural Practice

At medical school, our general practice attachment involved shadowing a GP for a month. Rather than simply shadow them at work, however, the medical school went full 'immersive theatre' – you had to actually live with them. Although it sounded like a reality TV experiment, stories I'd heard from students in other years made it seem like something of a minibreak. As well as learning undergraduate general practice, you got to travel to a different part of the country and stay in a lovely house, where a kindly spouse would help you stave off scurvy with some delicious home-cooked food. If you were lucky, you'd even have enough spare time to cram in lashings of revision. GP shadowing apparently also served as an incredible recruitment tool – previously flagging or aimless students would often begin to think, 'You know what, I could do this!'

When I mentioned to my dad that my GP placement was coming up, his face immediately switched to an expression I'd never seen before: pride, excitement and nostalgia in the same mixing bowl. He not-so-casually brought up the prospect of his retirement. It had never occurred to me over all those years I was being prepped and polished that I might follow in his footsteps so literally. Maybe that's the answer to everything – repeat history but try to make a slightly better job of it. I suppose that's what parenting is. I told myself that, for Dad, I'd give it my best shot.

Dr Pym was an incredible doctor. A proper old-school family GP who was only in his fifties but seemed somehow to belong to a bygone age. He knew every single one of his patients and could tell me their potted history well before Windows 95 could conjure up their notes. The patients adored him. Half of them would bring gifts to their appointments – homemade shortbreads and jams, misshapen gingerbread men baked by the adorable results of pregnancies he'd supervised, that sort of thing. His desk looked like a Comic Relief bake sale by the end of every day. As with GPs everywhere, however, the job had changed – patient numbers were up, and a surgery that used to have three doctors now only had two, ever since a clearly much-beloved colleague called Richard had moved on. In his absence, Dr Pym was forced to extend surgery hours earlier into the morning and later into the evening, then squeezed appointment times till they were well under the ten-minute mark. Soon the concept of a lunch break was entirely abandoned. I'd never seen anyone work harder. For nine hours straight, he'd face an onslaught of patients – person after person after person in one constant, unremitting stream of human need. Of course, one of a GP's most important skills is the spotting of the genuinely sick★ patient from the chaff who could be paracetamolled away. Unfortunately, it's a skill that becomes exponentially more difficult to perform the less time you have with someone,

---

★ 'Sick' is a medical term. It's short for 'really, really sick' and is often the first question a colleague will ask you about a patient: 'Are they sick?'

and at the conveyor-belt pace Dr Pym was expected to process his patients, it was bordering on impossible. His job had become like a lightning-speed version of Whack-a-Mole, with the added frisson that some of the moles might be malignant.

Dr Pym had the things he particularly enjoyed, such as psychiatry, dermatology, family planning, and the things he absolutely hated, such as muscles and joints (Richard always used to see to those, apparently). But I guess that's the same for every GP. You wouldn't know to watch him consult, though; every patient seemed to hold his utmost captive attention and the true magic trick was that no one – not even those with muscle or joint complaints – left his surgery feeling short-changed after their eight minutes. After closing time, he would alternate between staying back for a couple of hours to do paperwork and making house calls. (Richard always used to do a lot of the home visits, but now there were only two of them to share them out.)

Sadly, as far as my nutrition was concerned, his skills didn't extend to cooking and there was no Mr or Mrs Pym or matronly housekeeper to rustle me up a Linda McCartney sausage casserole. My dinner for the duration was either a Co-op cheese and onion sandwich (there was only one shop, which only sold one vegetarian sandwich) or a portion of chips from the chippy. I ate a lot of chips.

When we eventually returned home, Dr Pym didn't want to hang out on the sofa with me, shooting the breeze. Of course he didn't. I'd already been hanging around his periphery all day, lurking like some socially awkward vampire, soaking up his medical knowledge. Instead, when I walked in the front door at night, I'd take off my shoes and socks, put on a pair of handily provided disposable white socks and head upstairs to bed.

Ah yes. The socks.

Every doctor has their quirks. Niche interests, like miniature railways, scrapbooking or roadkill taxidermy. The demands of the job are such that many doctors need something external in which to immerse themselves, to escape into. Dr P's quirk – or at least the one that was most visible to me – was cleanliness, on a gargantuan scale. His house was so abnormally clean and tidy that it made a pathology lab look like a burger van's dustbin. He let it be known that these standards of cleanliness were to be scrupulously maintained; it was like living in a show home or sharing a house with Mr Sheen. There were almost no signs of human habitation beyond essential items such as chairs and beds – no photos, no ornaments, none of the usual detritus that people accumulate. I might have thought he was a spy but he plainly didn't have the time.

Besides, maybe it made sense for people to change into special house socks every evening? Sweaty day-worn socks really aren't that much better than shoes. Touching doors using only the handles made sense too – it's what they're there for! And while cleaning toilet bowl faecal smears by hand with a single sheet of loo roll took a small amount of getting used to, I reluctantly found myself agreeing that it was a more effective experience than prodding at them with a frazzled toilet brush. And as a guest in his house, who was I to argue? So I toed the line, and after seven hours' kip in my forensically scrubbed cell, it was back downstairs for a bowl of cereal eaten over the sink, then a quick wipe of the front door and off to work.

If it didn't tip into the realms of diagnosably compulsive behaviour, then perhaps the house rules were Dr P's way of establishing some degree of order in his life, in contrast to the relentless chaos of his job. And relentless really was the only word for it. When I imagined actually living his life, year in, year out, I felt a storm of panic swirling inside me.

I thought a lot about my dad. If Dr Pym coped with the pressures of the job by sandblasting every surface of his house with industrial-strength detergent, might my dad's quiet manner and carefully chosen paucity of words be a reflection of the work he did rather than, as I'd sometimes thought, because he wasn't hugely interested in us? Working for decades as a GP on a pretty unforgiving London estate must have taken up so much of his energy during the day that a dialled-down version of himself was all he could manage at home. GPs might leave their patients' notes at the surgery but the thoughts of what they've seen, patient after patient, must rattle round their head like pinballs.

Technically, we did have the option of going home at weekends, but as I couldn't afford the return train fare, I stayed. One Saturday morning, when Dr Pym had gone in to catch up on paperwork, I found myself left to my own devices. Worried I might leave a careless fingerprint on the toaster or accidentally shed too many skin cells, I decided to absent myself from the antiseptic nightmare of his house. I took a book of past exam papers to the beautiful village church and managed a couple of hours' work on a bench in the graveyard until the rows of tombstones with their stark reminder of the inevitability of death and the ultimate futility of medicine began to overwhelm me. Steering myself back from the edge of a modest existential calamity, I relocated to the pub, which was a lot lighter on explicit reminders of mortality and had the added advantage of trading in alcohol.

I found a dingy nook and continued to torture myself with exam questions over a soothing glass of bad white wine. The barman wandered over. 'Are you one of Dr Pym's lads?' I can't have been the first of his charges to seek refuge in the bottom of a glass. 'He's such a gentleman – you're lucky to have him as a teacher.'

He was right. Every day, I'd seen dozens more patients than I would have in any hospital setting and I'd started learning how to manage their hopes, fears and expectations with composure and kindness. When I went to the bar for another glass of wine, he wouldn't take my money. Instead, he handed me a bottle, which I nursed for a couple of hours before he brought me another. And then maybe another? The alcohol started to peel the edges from my reality and anaesthetise my doubts about medicine. I found myself seriously considering my life as a village GP.

Useful as med school had been for teaching me to handle my drink, my liver had its limits, and that day, with precisely 100 per cent of my calorific intake coming from Pinot Grigio, those limits had been exceeded. How far they'd been exceeded only really hit me once I'd tiptoed up to my bedroom in my regulation socks, stripped off my clothes and found myself clinging to a rapidly spinning bed. I tried to ignore it but as the night crawled on, my stomach began to insist that it was no longer the place for all the wine I'd consumed. The idea of vomiting was made about sixty times worse by the thought of having to do so in my boss's sterile show-pad. I wrestled against my gag reflex for a good hour or so, but once my retching had begun to toss the warning dribs of a spewnami into my mouth, I admitted defeat and urgently relocated to the bathroom.

In the small number of seconds during which I maintained control of my oesophagus, I played through the physics of the situation, like a snooker player approaching the baize. To ensure the bathroom remained unsullied, it was absolutely paramount that I avoided any splashback. I achieved this by ramming my head as deep into the bowl as possible. Not my finest hour, but it proved fairly effective when the first expulsion hit, as soon as fringe made contact with toilet-water. Being so close to the toilet bowl meant the splashback had literally nowhere to go, so my entire face was instantly coated with a mask of body temperature, bile-infused Jacob's Creek, some of which forced its way behind my horrified eyelids, but all of which stayed within the confines of the bowl. The encore, much less vicious, was easily contained within the porcelain. At this point, perhaps naïvely, I dared to feel the slightest wave of relief. Showing up maybe a minute later, however, the third wave was the strongest yet. It felt like every muscle, not just in my abdomen but in my entire body, had joined forces and tensed in unison, with the sole aim of propelling anything that wasn't physically attached to the inside of my body into the outside world. I took the position.

I hadn't, however, factored into my Newtonian calculations the possibility that all this straining and evacuation might also trigger some turbulence down the other end. It only actually occurred to me once the tradesman's revolt was well underway. Most of the diarrhoea came out in the first jet, spraying across the floor tiles behind me and tagging the deep plush pile of the super-absorbent snow-white fluffy bathmat. Wiping the vomit from my eyes, I glanced back at the carnage and felt genuine horror. Not since I was fourteen and saw my mother approaching with a handful of scrunched-up tissues from under my bed wondering if I 'had a cold' had I experienced such a combination of repulsion and panic. I knew I had to remove the bathmat from the bathroom and either get it dry cleaned or incinerated and replaced with another, before the good doctor found out.

And so it was that Dr Pym, either disturbed by the noise or leaving his bedroom to perform some night-time ablution or other, saw me creeping across his landing, buck naked and bleary-eyed, his once pristine bathmat held tightly to my chest, so that no more of my poop-soup could defile his house.

As any psychology professional will tell you, it's good to get things out in the open and engage in honest, direct dialogue – it's just the healthy way. Sometimes, however, it's better to bottle it up and pretend certain things never happened at all, which is handily how most doctors deal with their issues, and the route Dr Pym and I both tacitly chose for the remainder of my attachment.

And as we slogged through the rest of our time together, the pace of Dr Pym's working days never let up – it was like watching an endurance athlete cycling the Sahara. Tougher than that, in truth, as he was never going to run out of desert and hit the Red Sea; the patients would just keep coming, until the end of time.

At our debrief session, Dr Pym took a genuine interest in my career and had a lot of questions – thankfully none of them related to the bathmat. I also had questions for him. I was curious as to why they hadn't replaced Richard.

He laughed. They'd been trying for two years, he said, but couldn't find anyone who wanted to work in the middle of Nowhere St Bullshit for the kind of money that was on offer. 'So, what's the plan?' I asked. 'Keep going like this until you die from a heart attack at your desk?'

'I don't see why not,' he said. 'It worked for Richard.'

Chapter 8

Despite having a day or two of diffuse lower abdominal pain, I decided not to hector my GP about it – it was probably just trapped wind or some kind of stress ulcer caused by moving house twice in eighteen months. Either way, it would probably sort itself out before I'd managed to 'press four for an appointment within the next ten years' on the medical centre's tangled phone tree. Besides, I was in my thirties – any car that age would have a few weird rattles and warning lights by then, nothing to think too much about. J, however, wasn't interested in my automotive analogies, other than threatening to brain me with a lug wrench if I didn't seek medical attention. I reminded him that I spent six years at med school and many more on the wards and he reminded me about what happened in Las Vegas.★ He would sooner take Dr Dre or Dr Pepper's opinion over mine.

I came up with a compromise: I would call my dad and ask for his advice. J thought this was sensible because I'd be getting the benefit of a GP with decades of experience. I thought this was sensible because, knowing my dad, there was a roughly

---

★ Totally forgetting that what happens in Las Vegas stays in Las Vegas.

zero per cent chance he would tell me to bother a doctor. Growing up, every single emergency was handled in-house, from concussions ('Where there's no sense, there's no feeling') to gaping wounds ('Not much jam') – I got through an entire school career without ever being granted a morning off sick. I have a scar on my forehead to this day from one particular homespun, in retrospect slightly ham-fisted, repair of a head injury and I'm sure that had the situation arisen, he would've given an organ transplant a bash too.

At J's insistence, I put my dad on speakerphone – my Vegas behaviour had dented his trust slightly – and, true to form, he told me it would probably settle down in a couple of days and to call him if it didn't. It didn't.★

That evening, while innocently conducting my business at a pub urinal, my urine turned from a healthy beery blond to an alarming shade of claret. The horrified face of my neighbour at the trough strongly implied that, were it his urinary tract,

---

★ In fairness to him, most things *do* settle down. At medical school, we learned about a doctor called Archie Cochrane. While serving in the British Army in Crete in 1941, he was captured by the Nazis and found himself holed up in a prisoner-of-war camp where they appointed him chief medical officer and put him in charge of the hospital. Technically, it wasn't much of a hospital, as it contained none of the things a hospital normally contains, like doctors, nurses and medical supplies. When people were admitted to the hospital, as they frequently were, Cochrane would ask the Nazis for medical supplies, to which they would reply '*Ärtze sind überflüssig*' – 'Doctors are superfluous'. But I guess they were a famously unsympathetic bunch, the Nazis. Unable to actually treat his patients, Cochrane simply documented their symptoms and monitored their progress, realising in the process that, at least as far as doctors were concerned, the Nazis may have had a point. It seemed that doctors really were, if not exactly superfluous, then at least far less necessary than previously imagined. Archie's book, *Effectiveness and Efficiency: Random Reflections on Health Services* was published in 1972 and was hugely influential in advocating for randomised trials when testing treatments. Didn't sell as many as mine, though.

he would definitely seek medical attention. But I decided there was still no need – I had a diagnosis: a bladder stone floating around in my piss, and all I had to do was wait to see if it passed. If it didn't, I would begrudgingly bother the NHS, but in the meantime, I would pursue a policy of watchful waiting.* Over the next twenty-four hours, the stone was definitely on the move and had found its way out of my bladder, and was slowly millimetring its way down the length of my penis.

Despite having witnessed more than my fair share, I wouldn't presume to know what childbirth feels like, but I can at least more closely empathise with the concept of having an oversized object squeezing its way down an eye-wateringly ill-prepared genital tract at the pace of a queue for the Nemesis on a bank holiday Monday. It's remarkably difficult to describe pain, which is why doctors ask you to rate it out of ten or, if you're a child (or you look like you haven't yet mastered numbers all the way up to ten), point to the cutesy emoji that best reflects what you're feeling. The emoji I required was yet to be dreamed up by the designers but it would have probably needed a speech bubble saying 'THERE'S A STONE STUCK IN MY COCK AND I'M PISSING BLOOD!'

The stone needed to be flushed out, so I spent a day drinking absurd quantities of water to help it on its way. Simple physics. Litres and litres of drinking and pissing and drinking and pissing and . . . nothing: it was wedged, like a child's head in the bannisters. That evening, I tried a different tack: I carried on drinking but stopped pissing. I figured that if I held it in for a couple of hours, I'd be able to generate enough pressure

---

* Or as J less charitably referred to it, 'stupid ignoring'.

to just blast the thing out. Like a ghostbuster. All I actually managed to do was somehow rotate the stone into an even more agonising position.

Writhing around in bed at 2 a.m., I toyed briefly with the idea of using the syringe I de-wax my ears with to squirt the stone back up to the relative comfort of my bladder. By 4 a.m., I was wondering if maybe I could construct some kind of sufficiently small grabber device, like at a fairground arcade – except I'd be winning a urine-soaked pebble instead of a teddy bear. A crocodile clip would *just about* get up there, at a painful push – but opening it would probably be impossible and I'd doubtless find myself as some surgeon's latest dinner party anecdote: the guy with the crocodile clip in his cock.

By 7 a.m., I realised the problem with my earlier physics experiment: urine is simply too thin a liquid to dislodge a stone. What I needed was some kind of freezing wand, which I could wave over my bladder, generating tiny ice bullets. Peeing out these frozen pellets would bombard the stone and set it, and me, free. I searched the internet: surely such a thing existed in the worlds of catering, agriculture or perverts? Sadly not. With time against me, I had to rule out an appearance on *Dragons' Den* to raise finance for my invention. Then it hit me. While my useless body couldn't produce ice, it could produce something more viscous than urine.

You don't often hear people talk about their worst wank. Worst birthday, worst car, worst date, sure, but not worst wank. I suppose some amongst us might remember the time their parents walked in on them, or the time they sprained their wrist, or crashed their car. Certainly, were he able to communicate from the afterlife, Michael Hutchence would have a story that would be difficult to beat. My worst wank was an agonising twenty-minute affair, trying to ejaculate while every stroke felt like I was grating my cock from the inside using a rasp. As turn-ons go, it was up there with watching my parents fuck *their* parents in a Berlin scat club.★ Somehow, through sheer desperation, I was able to pull on the full depths of my inner resources and finish the job. I guess I expected an eruption to rival Vesuvius, for the stone to shoot out as if it was bound for Goliath's head, and for all my pain to be instantly relieved. I even made sure it wasn't pointing towards the window. As it happened . . . nothing happened. No stone, no sperm, nothing. Instead, I'd managed to cause some kind of logjam – it was like trying to shoot birthday cake out of a water pistol.

I lay across the back seat as J drove me to Charing Cross Hospital, muttering angrily to himself that he fucking knew he shouldn't have listened to me in the first place. I felt like I was in some kind of X-rated Aesop's fable about why you should always go to the doctor sooner rather than later. Of course I knew what would happen next: a urologist,† inevitably some fuckball I'd previously worked with, would stick a thick metal scope inside me and the stone would spurt out on a tsunami of cum, piss and blood – a horrible hodgepodge of everything my penis has ever produced. Bright side: I was in with a fair chance of winning the Turner Prize.

I walked up to the A&E front desk. Name, address, date of birth. Without even thinking, I announced myself as Dr Adam Kay. After all, I was a doctor in name – I still had the degree certificate somewhere. There must have been a part of me that thought I might get treated a little more favourably. Maybe

---

★   This is a metaphor, not a memory.

†   Another famously unsympathetic bunch.

I'd even skip the queue, like a competition winner at Thorpe Park.

I limped to the toilets in the A&E waiting room. In a stained cubicle that smelled like a sewer-worker's verucca sock,★ the universe took pity on me and my body managed an eleventh-hour reprieve: my beleaguered penis hoicked up the stone all by itself. To say that I was disappointed by the size of my tormentor is an understatement. I was expecting a barbed-wire pineapple. Instead, it was more like something you might scrape from your eye in the morning. That didn't matter. What mattered was, it was gone, and I was free.

I caught up with my dad that weekend. 'How's the tummy ache?'

'Yep, sorted itself out.'

'What did I say?'

★   This is a memory, not a metaphor.

– FLASHBACK –

Famously Unsympathetic

As a medical student, I must have been asked at least three hundred times, 'What kind of doctor are you going to be?' It came from all angles: bumping into second-degree relatives at weddings and connecting with old schoolmates on FriendsReunited on my Evesham Micros Voyager 2000.* Of course, at the time, I had no idea. Apart from the occasional eye pervert who'd known from the age of five that they were destined to be an ophthalmologist, no one at medical school had any kind of plan beyond scraping through the yearly exams and, if at all possible, not dying in a drinking game.

But every placement I went on ruled out another specialty as a potential career path. Like a slightly bilious game of Guess Who?, I'd already excluded general

---

* Ignore this footnote if you're old enough to think a catfish is something that swims in the river rather than a fifty-eight-year-old data entry clerk from Godalming. FriendsReunited was a pre-Facebook where you would register your school and year of graduation, and be served up with details of former classmates and how much happier and more successful they were than you. My mother now offers a very similar service.

practice, followed by haematology, then orthopaedics.*
My next potential suitor was urology.

I arrived on the ward, my short white coat freshly ironed
and my eyes canyon-wide in wonderment at the possi-
bilities yawning before me. My Mr Miyagi was a young
registrar called Peter who, sadly, saw me less as the Karate
Kid and more as some kind of large bipedal tumour.

Peter suffered from a debilitating condition that meant
his internal monologue was wired up to an amp. When,
for example, I introduced myself as his medical student,
he yelled, 'Oh, for fuck's sake!' Then he despatched me
to A&E to clerk a couple of patients who were waiting for
urology review.

The problem with clinical attachments is that the person
charged with teaching you is a junior doctor, and junior
doctors are not renowned for having copious amounts of
spare time. So, just as a bothersome toddler might be compelled by an end-of-tether parent to go count the blades
of grass on the lawn, a medical student may be sent off by
the junior doctor to clerk a patient.†

---

* I ended up in obs and gynae through a casserole of misapprehensions. Thanks
to watching too many Lenor ads, I quite liked the idea of being around newborn
babies, which turn out to be cute the first ... maybe three times, I suppose? Plus
there was the idea that the job was straightforward. It was, practically – cut here,
pull there, stitch here, wrap this in a towel – but it wasn't emotionally. Not on the
bad shifts.

† Clerking is the first assessment a patient undergoes – a long list of questions
and a rudimentary physical examination, leading ideally to a plan of management.
Patients often forget key details when being interrogated by a medical student.
I'm sure it's down to the stress of the situation or not realising which details might
be important – but for the student it often feels like you're in some kind of hidden
camera show, where you're being made to look catastrophically inept. I get how
someone might neglect to mention she's taking an oral contraceptive because it's

I asked Peter if he'd prefer me to present the patients one at a time or after I'd seen them both. Peter informed me that there was nothing in the entire universe that could possibly interest him less and I smiled, as graciously as I could manage. The fact was, I needed Peter's signature of approval at the end of this placement, so I had no option other than to lap it up. I lapped, then headed down to A&E.

My place in the hierarchy was cemented when the first patient I introduced myself to also greeted me with an inducement to fuck right off. In fairness, he'd been promised an expert review and was being presented with the direct opposite of that. I eventually got him on side by saying that a quick chat with me would get him to the front of the queue to see my boss. Technically a lie but a credible one, plus it worked, and nobody died. As I wasn't in much of a hurry to be flame-grilled by Peter, I sat down for an hour and studiously recorded his story. I channelled my inner Letterman, asking as many vaguely relevant questions as I could muster.

'I would suggest,' I eventually told him, 'that the reason you've been unable to pass urine is . . . ' I paused, like I was about to reveal the top prize in a tombola or unmask the killer in an ITV drama '. . . because of the tramadol you've been taking for your back pain.' I clearly had an innate aptitude for urology – the wand had chosen the wizard on my very first placement. Remarkable!

I wasn't exactly expecting to be showered in glitter or for the patient to struggle to a standing ovation, but

---

such a forgettably routine occurrence, but I can't quite understand the mental blip that led a patient to tell me they had no significant medical history, before revealing to the consultant that they'd actually had a kidney transplant, for which they took a daily handbagful of drugs.

I had hoped for rather more than a shrug and an 'And?'
He wanted to know what we were going to do about it. I
confessed that I had absolutely no idea but I'd return shortly
with my registrar, who absolutely would. In rather inele-
gant terms, the patient made it clear that he considered our
entire interaction a diabolical waste of time. It was hard to
disagree.

The second patient, on the other hand, seemed extremely pleased to see me. I couldn't take full credit for his
erection, however. Most of that had to go to the Viagra
he'd necked the night before.* He began to suspect that
something might be amiss when his morning glory continued well past his Weetabix and became a right pain in the
cock. When he sought medical advice, he got me. Neither
of us seemed especially thrilled with the arrangement.
Like a Poirot of the penis, I made the diagnosis instantly:
priapism – the medical term for an erection that overstays
its welcome. Then, snapping on a pair of surgical gloves
and my very best poker face, I said, 'I should probably
examine . . . it.' It was shortly thereafter, with this stubby
but forthright seventy-five-year-old erection pulsing

---

* Prior to Viagra, or sildenafil to use its drag name, the alchemy of turning
blancmange into rock was dominated by prosthetic devices that were inserted
into the penis and activated with a couple of careful squeezes of a rubber ball hidden inside the scrotum. Sexy, for sure, but in the heat of the moment not quite as
handy as a little blue pill. Drug-wise, Viagra was preceded by phenoxybenzamine,
the success of which was severely limited by the fact that it needed to be injected. In order to demonstrate the efficacy of phenoxybenzamine to the American
Urological Association, Dr Giles Brindley whipped out his bloated johnson and
invited his assembled colleagues in a packed lecture hall to examine it. Remarkably, none of them called the police. Dr Brindley also once appeared on *Tomorrow's
World* to demonstrate a new type of bassoon he had invented. If he whipped his
cock out on this occasion, it didn't make the final cut.

between my forefingers, that I was confidently able to rule out urology as my career path.*

I wrote up my notes in the canteen with its bizarre pricing system that meant you were always carrying spare change with you in the afternoon. I ate a £3.61 jacket potato and jangled back upstairs to present my findings to my registrar. I began with Tramadol Man and, with his feet up on the nursing station, Peter nodded along to my story, peppering his seeming lack of interest with snide remarks and unpleasantries generally reserved for one's inside voice. He was to be catheterised and sent up to the ward. Fine. Then came the headliner. 'This is Mr Fury, a seventy-five-year-old retired blacksmith, who presents with a nine-hour episode of priapism secondary to the use of sildenafil.'

Peter jumped to his feet. 'Where is he now?'

'Down in A&E,' I replied.

'That's a urological emergency, you fucking cretin. Why didn't you call me?'

Because you're about as approachable as a far-right Rottweiler with gum disease? I tried to keep up with Peter as he pelted down to A&E. Barely three hours in the building and I'm picturing the GMC hearing where I get struck off before I'm even qualified. Watching the trial is an incredulous panel of jurors, gasping as they hear how I merrily ate a jacket potato while, thanks to my wilful inaction, a man's entire genitalia dissolved into a gorgonzola fondue. I spluttered my excuses as we got into A&E but Peter couldn't have given less of a shit. I directed him towards the cubicle

---

* As it turned out, I had no say in the matter and was allocated urology in my first year as a doctor. Still, I got a lot of anecdotes out of it and dinner parties would never be the same again.

and he whooshed open the curtain to reveal a middle-aged woman with a shocked expression, but no erection.

Peter looked at me with all the affection of an abattoir stun gun and a nurse explained that the urology patient had discharged himself, his erection having subsided of its own accord shortly after coming into contact with me. Feelings of relief that both my career and the patient would live to see another day were matched by the slight dent of pride that I'd caused such an instantaneous cock-shrinking with my magic hands.

Peter shoved past me, pausing only to bark 'Fucking timewaster' over his shoulder. I skulked in place as an entire A&E department witnessed my humiliation. I breathed it in and readied myself for the next round. Teaching by humiliation. Teaching by bullying. That's just how it is in medicine, and how it's always been. It's seen as a necessary evil, perpetuated by visibly harmed doctors who say, 'It never did me any harm.' Or worse still, ones who are unaware that they're doing it. I'm not sure what's worse – that I ended up doing it to medical students myself or that not a single person pulled me up on it because it's so deeply entrenched in the culture of medical education. Doctors need to be toughened up to deal with the hell of the job, and medical school is on hand to make that happen.

However, one man's necessary evil is another, nicer man's totally unnecessary evil. Perhaps one day, the compassion and empathy that should flow freely from doctors to patients will be a perfect reflection of the compassion and empathy that flows downstream in hospitals and medical schools. But not today. In the meantime, I hope Peter eventually finds a position more suited to his particular set of skills, such as torture garden operative or home secretary.

Chapter 9

A text from H, out of the blue. Ambrose was ill.

Ambrose had first appeared in the final months of our time together – that age-old trick of bringing in a sentient being to plaster over a relationship crack. He was a tiny ball of irrepressible kitteny fluff with a party trick of running up and down my piano keyboard, playing scales like he was in a Bisney film. When we split up, there wasn't really a case for him living with me – I was in a bit of a state mentally, financially and residentially; my bank manager and houseplants would have been in unanimous agreement that taking on any kind of responsibility would have been a profoundly bad idea – so he went to live with H. He was still technically 'our' cat, but I found my visiting rights too painful to exercise, so I drifted into the role of absent parent, no better than the 'bad dads' who eventually tire of spending their Sundays in a draughty McDonald's watching their estranged progeny push Chicken McNuggets around the box.

I idly wondered if he missed me, whether he ever stopped to think why he hadn't seen me stubbing my toe on his litter tray recently or where the piano had gone. But I didn't cut off contact altogether: he would still come to stay with me when H was off on holiday. And I kept paying the insurance – the triple-extra-platinum cover, because there's no feline version of the NHS and nothing was too good for Ambrose, wherever he lived.

And now he needed me. A vet visit had revealed that one of his kidneys was very dilated; far more dilated, in fact, than this high-street practice knew how to deal with. They suggested, therefore, that Ambrose be taken to specialist veterinary surgeons, who might be able to operate on his kidney and save his life.

This specialist hospital was a good sixty-mile drive away, so we drove out together, with me at the wheel, H in the passenger seat and Ambrose in his cage, strapped to the backseat. At one point, I praised him for being so quiet and behaving so well – normally he wouldn't shut the fuck up in the car – realising as I said it that . . . of course he's quiet; he's too sick to make any kind of fuss.

Although the circumstances weren't particularly ideal, our drive to the cat hospital gave rise to the longest chat we'd had for years and I was glad for it. It was nice to have the time to properly catch up. Seeing an ex after a break-up is a bit like coming back after a gap year. You look each other up and down; everything is still where it used to be; they're the same person, but there are hints of the personal evolution that happened since you left each other's lives. Gradually, you become almost unrecognisable to one another and it's impossible to even imagine that you'd ever bickered over who ate the last Kinder Bueno.* We were the very picture of exes behaving well, politely enquiring after one another's replacement paramours, holidays planned and friends we'd lost in the split

---

* It was H.

– none of the fierce chill of the final throes. Our mutual respect for Ambrose, and for each other's relationship with Ambrose, insulated us from the cold.

I felt sick with worry as I carried Ambrose in his cage across the car park, fast-walking in case the extra four seconds I saved might make all the difference. My breathing was shallow and uneven, anxious at taking the little fellow into the unknown.

And then something changed as I walked through the double doors – it wasn't unknown any more, it was Proustian and familiar. Staff in white coats and tunics, pagers bleeping, the smell of disinfectant and all that it masks, the air of carefully constructed calm. A nurse came to take Ambrose and I gave a few unnecessary sentences of handover in medicalese. I don't know why. Maybe it's the mother tongue I automatically revert to in a medical environment. Maybe I reckoned my vague air of knowledgeability might make them take extra care of him. Maybe I was just comforting myself by trying to feel some control in a situation where I had none.

Me and H sat in the foyer and I postured about what they'd be doing now – putting in drips and taking blood. Presumably they'd have to shave his legs for that: it's hard enough putting drips into humans and they're not covered in thick orange fur.

A sign on the wall pointed to the horse surgery unit and the blood bank. I shared my mental image of a massive horse lying on a gigantic bed and hooked up to a binbag full of blood. H smiled. Humour – my armour and my weakness. It was certainly being tested that day.

Those staff walking by – some of them must have been looking after Ambrose. What did they know that we didn't? I remembered making that same slow walk across to a hopeful face, trying to keep my own as composed and unreadable as I could, practising my lines to make sure they came out kindly, clearly, authoritatively. Would I be met with nodding acceptance, stifled cries, deep breaths or racking sobs?

H snapped me back into the moment, asking if I was alright. 'Yep. Fine.'

An hour later, a bescrubbed vet appeared to explain that Ambrose had been admitted to intensive care and that they'd re-image him in the morning with a view to putting a stent inside his swollen kidney. I cracked a joke about a cat scan. H didn't react and the vet made it quite clear it wasn't the first time he'd heard that joke, probably not even the first time that day. 'Is he going to live?' I asked, and the vet gave a qualified yes – his bloods needed to stabilise a little overnight but there was no reason to think the stent wouldn't do the job. H choked up and grabbed my hand. I thanked the vet calmly, bordering on stiffly, and said it sounded very reassuring. I was elated, obviously, but I was in a hospital for god's sake and that's no place for emotions.

The return journey was a slightly cheerier affair, as we both allowed ourselves to relax a little and drop some of our earlier formality. By the time I deposited H back, we'd even managed to launch a couple of appropriately cattish digs at each other, which was nice and comfortable. Like old times.

The next day, H updated me. Ambrose had had a good night and they were more optimistic than ever about a full recovery after surgery. There was, however, a tiny spanner in the works. The treatment was going to cost £6,000 and the insurance people – doers of utter evil that they are – were refusing to cover a penny of it.★

The simple truth was that neither of us had that kind of money. Not even close. I'd sunk all my savings and spoils from grim best man speeches into two slugs of stamp duty; I had a job with the stability of an Argos shelving unit and a bank balance that barely covered the tank of petrol which took us to the hospital. The insurers stuck to their heartless guns, despite phone call after begging phone call. The only other option – aside from the six-grand operation – was to put Ambrose to sleep. As a gesture of goodwill, stretching the word 'goodwill' until it broke into a thousand poisonous pieces, the insurers offered to fund Ambrose's murder, as well as having brought it about.

On my second journey back from the hospital I was accompanied by a small cardboard box marked 'Ambrose Kay'. I could only assume the bizarre addition of my surname was intended to hammer the guilt home further. This poor little cat, I felt so desperately sorry for him. When I took him on, it was a promise to look after him – even if it did end up being on a timeshare basis. He provided me with unconditional love and the occasional dead rodent, and I let him down. I felt for H, who must have had it far worse – I didn't even live with the cat. I felt sorry for the vet, who surely never imagined

---

★ Had I read the policy? Yes, I'd looked at the main points when I took it out. Had I read every last sentence of the deliberately obfuscatory fineprint? Of course not, no one does. Then, a few years later, they jump up out of the smallprint and stab you in the heart. In size two microfiche font, hidden among an old testament's worth of legal bullshit and intricate tripwires of specific wording, a maximum payment clause whispered about the total amount that could be paid out for a single condition and, with just a couple of vet visits and a handful of antibiotics, we had apparently already exceeded it. Insurers are criminally-adjacent fuckpieces and the only thing separating them from mafiosi is headed notepaper.

when signing up for vet school that one day she might have to put three-year-old animals to sleep because their owners were simply too poor to let them live. *Sophie's Choice* it clearly wasn't but I loved that cat, and it was my fault he died.

The horrible truth was that if I hadn't jacked in medicine, I'd have probably been able to scrape the money together – another reason to feel guilty about leaving, on top of the patients and colleagues I'd let down and the effort that was wasted on my training.

But this was different. A living creature was dead. Or maybe it wasn't so different – who knows the life and death implications of yet another doctor missing from the rota. Who the hell did I think I was? By putting myself first, it was only natural that everyone else in my universe had to move down a rank – and poor Ambrose had been edged off the leader board altogether.

We scattered Ambrose's ashes around his favourite tree in the garden of H's flat. I didn't know Ambrose had a favourite tree, but I could imagine him scampering up the trunk. Not too high though – he didn't like heights that much. I was glad that Ambrose had got to live here: a nice flat with a nice garden, and was only slightly pissed off how much nicer it was than my new flat.

We shared memories of Ambrose, mine a lot more distant than H's. H was clearly upset and I dealt with it all a lot better. By which I mean I dealt with it a lot worse by pretending I was fine. We hugged, said our goodbyes and promised to keep in touch, even though the last practical reason to do so was nothing more than ashes round a tree. I started the drive home and then a warning light came on. Not in the car – I ignore those – but in the form of a choking sob somewhere in my throat. A stiff upper lip malfunction. I pulled into the Texaco on Wandsworth Road and cried everything out of me. It took about twenty minutes. I reset my face and started the engine.

Chapter 10

My leg had started hurting. Badly. Bolts of electricity were flashing down my calf dozens of times a day. I could even pinpoint the exact nerve root in my back that was causing it – not because of any great skill in neurology, more because my previous operation was in that exact place. I also knew precisely what my spinal surgeon would say if I went back to him because he'd previously told me what he'd need to do should symptoms recur. The next operation would involve not just scalpels and discs, but also metal rods and the fusing of vertebrae. Godsake.

Obviously after penis-stone-gate there was no way I could tell J this was happening – he'd have me straight back to spinal clinic, subjected to hours of invasive fuckery and months of re-covery. If he caught me wincing, I would say that I'd stubbed my toe or had a migraine. Unable to moan at home, the agony erupted from me during a lunch break while I was working on a TV show.* One of the other writers, Carol, said, 'Oh, I had that exact same pain. I saw this osteopath who sorted it right out.'

---

* I thought the programme was pretty solid but viewers disagreed, staying away in their droves. Ratings are rounded to the nearest 50,000 people, and this show registered zero.

Maybe it's because of my training in conventional medicine or maybe it's because my IQ is higher than that of a skirting board, but I've never been a huge fan of alternative medicine. If a new therapy comes along – whether it's cutting-edge immunotherapy or plonking hot stones on someone's back like you're laying a rock garden – you do a study. If it works, you call it medicine. If it doesn't work, you put it in the bin and try something else. Somehow, a whackjob third way has wormed itself in, whereby if something is proven not to work but has enough mindless devotees, then it gets declared 'alternative medicine' and if you call it out for being nonsense, you're just narrow-minded.

What is it an alternative to, exactly? Staying alive? Getting better? I understand that some people feel let down by conventional medicine (treatments that have been researched, proven to work and administered by qualified practitioners) and seek out another way (lake water dosed out by a liar in a tabard). Medicine might not have anything like all the answers, but at least it's prepared to show you its working.

Even a harmless treatment can be harmful: pissing about with sage-burning, runes and a two-pronged stick delays actual, useful treatment. I remember one patient in fertility clinic who had spent so long consulting her homeopathist that by the time she called it a day and opted for non-alternative medicine, she had tipped out of the eligible age range for IVF. Still, I'm sure all that water kept her well hydrated.

But Carol made a convincing case. 'It worked for me!' is surprisingly persuasive when you're in Dignitas-googling agony, with your vertebrae conspiring to grind flour in your spinal column. My sleep-deprived, liquefied brain began to power down its rational side. I wanted the pain to fuck off (rational), I didn't want to see a doctor (semi-rational, leaning towards irrational) and now there was the option of forty-five minutes on a pine-effect bench handing over a reassuringly nauseating amount of money to a kindly wizard (patently irrational). I took his number.

I sat in the waiting room and filled out my details on a clipboard, including a section about my aims and expectations. I kept quiet about my expectations. Checking over my details, a man in a white polo shirt asked me what kind of doctor I was. Maybe he suspected I was working undercover and was going to steal his best magic tricks for the NHS. I didn't fancy a scrap so I said I was a doctor of physics, then spent the whole session with my back more tense than ever, worrying he'd ask me literally anything about physics.*

I lay down on the bench and white polo man told me that I was so far out of alignment that he thought the pain in my leg might be coming from my shoulder, so that's what he'd work on initially. Tempted though I was to correct him with a quick rendition of 'The leg bone's not connected to the shoulder bone', I let him fiddle and footle with the totally wrong part of my body. Even if all I got from this was the placebo effect, that was enough for me.†

'What's your blood type?' asked the osteopath. 'A negative,' I replied. Was he going to . . . operate on me? No, he just wanted to ask about my diet, which was apparently somehow

---

* The only physics fact I can remember is that atoms are 99.loadsof9s per cent empty space, to the extent that if you took all of the actual matter that makes up the entire human race it would squish down to the size of a sugar cube.

† You don't need to believe in a placebo for it to work. Amazingly, even if you tell someone that you're giving them sugar pills for their condition and put them in a big box that says 'LITERALLY M&Ms', then they still enjoy the placebo effect.

incompatible with my blood type and might be throwing my spine out. Still, I was enjoying the massage, more or less. And anyway, who's to say the treatment might not genuinely work? Sure, there isn't any evidence today but who knows what the future holds? Maybe I was simply the bloke who Alexander Fleming persuaded to lick mould off a plate before the results came back from the trial.

Glancing at a patch of eczema on my arm, the osteopath then suggested that if he had time after he'd fixed my leg, a little cranial osteopathy would probably sort that out too. I smiled and nodded, like when one of my friends invites me to swipe through 700 photos of their kitchen rebuild. I held my tongue, closed my eyes and let him babble away about how traditional doctors don't really understand neurology.

He asked me when I first had problems with my back, and then gasped at my answer and stopped massaging. 'Well, you know what caused it then?' Oh god, no, what? The finale of *Lost*? West Ham appointing Avram Grant? Nope. 'That's when they turned on the Large Hadron Collider.'

I stood up, pulled myself together and thanked him for his time. Then, politely declaring that I needed to be elsewhere, by which I meant reality, I left his office feeling like a bloody idiot for ever having gone there in the first place. However, as I sprinted down the stairs, shaking my head and grumbling to myself, I have to say my leg was feeling substantially better . . .

Chapter 11

It occurred to me that an increasing number of my interactions with J were becoming irksome. Nothing extreme, nothing to panic about, there was just a slight exasperation creeping in. It was something that clearly required constructive and appropriate action to stop it getting any worse. Couple's counselling was obviously an option, but I couldn't shake the thought that I'd end up feeling like an audience member at a one-man West End show called *Fuck Adam*. No, I could work this out myself – I was a trained problem solver, after all. So I kept a mental note of every squabble and bicker to see if any patterns emerged.

It didn't take long before I hit my eureka moment: our arguments invariably began with me asking, as politely and calmly as Jesus himself would have done, why J had once again failed to uphold his half of the cleaning rota. J, tragically, was born without the part of the brain that allows him to apologise, so would respond by bringing up some incident from years ago, such as when one minute into a flight, I 'over-reacted' when J spilled a huge glass of orange juice onto my crotch.* And then

---

* J asked me to change this to say it was actually a member of cabin crew who spilled the orange juice and, when I refused to, didn't speak to me for a full twenty-four hours.

we'd scream at one another for a while, before I'd eventually storm off and sleep on the sofa. But of course the sofa was cold and not quite long enough, so I'd lie there in a combination of fury, hypothermia and intractable neck pain until I could hear him snoring, then I'd creep back to bed like a guilty dog. I presented J with a root-cause solution: I would arrange a cleaner. (And he would pay for them.)

I found Wanda on Gumtree, where she described herself as 'PERFECT CLEANER'. How could I not employ her? She was in her sixties, with the physique of a stickman drawn with a mechanical pencil. She was strong – extraordinarily strong – able to move wardrobes with minimal effort. She seemed to derive this strength from the pack of cigarettes she smoked in the flat over the course of the three hours a fortnight that she cleaned for us. Very quickly she began to feel like a member of the family, by which I mean she showed every outward sign of hating me and limited our interactions to the bare minimum.

On her second visit, I came home to find her cutting up my t-shirts, like a jilted lover in a soap opera.

'Is everything . . . OK?' I stuttered.

'I need to use them for cloths,' she explained. 'You can't wear these. It's embarrassing.'

I offered to get her the very finest cloths that money could buy, but she shook her head, ash tumbling from the cigarette dangling from her mouth and onto the carpet.

By the end of her fifth visit, everything in the flat had moved. Some ornaments had been rearranged on shelves and mantelpieces; some had been relegated entirely and hidden away in a box. The contents of every kitchen drawer and cupboard shelf had been allocated a new position. Even the sofas had been moved. 'It's better,' she stated flatly, leaving no room for discussion. 'You'll see.' We didn't see, but we couldn't face fighting with her: she was much stronger than us emotionally. Also, physically: we couldn't have moved the furniture back if we'd tried. All a bit irritating but . . . the arguments had stopped.

After a few months in our service, Wanda informed me she was happy to continue working for us. We'd clearly been on some kind of probation period without even realising.

'Thank you?' I replied.

'So ungrateful,' she said.

As the months ground on, she seemed to start warming to us. She took to calling me Adarsh, which she said was a term of endearment in Polish, but smiled knowingly when she said it, as if she was calling me a cunt to my face. One day, she picked up a letter addressed to 'Dr Adam Kay' and asked me how I could be a doctor when I never did any work. 'Doctor of what? Sitting on your arse?' When I explained that I was a former doctor, she scowled. She then told me it was disgraceful to leave a job like that, putting into a few words what my mother had thus far only managed to disguise in coded questions about how my 'little break' was working out.

But now the catheter was out of the bag, I could see Wanda's interest had been piqued. Perhaps she wanted me to help dispose of some bodies for her. She began to quiz me more closely. What was my specialty? 'Labour ward – delivering babies.' At which point, rather than the standard cooing or questions as to how many babies I'd delivered, she shook her head, told me I was disgusting and went off to snort a line of cumin (something she did regularly for her 'sinuses'). Her subsequent questions were generally quite dark and very rarely failed to surprise me. Did I ever slip with a scalpel during an operation? How much blood can a patient lose and still live?*

Once she even asked, 'Did you ever kill anyone?'

I laughed nervously as a flip book of everything that ever went wrong at work flashed before my eyes and I desperately searched for a joke to launch this conversation out of the danger zone.

'Never on purpose!'

'That's stupid joke, not answer,' she replied.

Another nervous laugh from me, another layer of fortified steel clanking into place. 'I could tell you, but I'd have to kill you too.'

'Always with the stupid joke.'

I don't know why I told this to Wanda – maybe the fact that she'd seen through me and called out my deflection. Perhaps the distance between us gave it a degree of anonymity, like a confession to a priest or a blowjob through a glory hole. Or alternatively, because I knew she'd have never stopped asking me until I did.

I told her about a man in his seventies who I killed as a junior doctor. I misread a microbiology report and prescribed him an antibiotic that his sepsis was resistant to rather than responsive to. My mistake was spotted the day afterwards but he got sicker and sicker and died a couple of weeks later. You could point to the other weak points in the chain which allowed this to happen: the pharmacist who didn't spot my error, my supervisors who weren't supervising. You could say that twenty-four hours on the wrong antibiotics wouldn't have made any difference. But you couldn't say that with absolute certainty. *Sliding*

---

* About a third of it, but please don't conduct any experiments.

Doors meets *ER*: if I hadn't made a mistake, he might have lived. It was the first time I'd said this out loud – the first time I'd said anything like this out loud – and I was saying it to a near stranger.

A problem shared isn't necessarily a problem halved. I didn't feel relief, I felt sick. Saying the words seemed to exhume and unlock every awful feeling I had back then, the lens of time somehow managing to magnify them. Maybe it's better to keep these memories buried in the bunker where you interred them.

Annoyingly, yet entirely predictably, Wanda much preferred J to me. Her son was gay, she told him, and although Poland sounded like a much tougher place to come out than England, she said it made her happy that he might one day end up with someone nice like J. He took the compliment in his stride, telling her she was very sweet and assuring her that her son would be fine. 'Hopefully not someone like him,' she continued, practically spitting towards the living room where I was sat.

One day, I came home to find Wanda in floods of tears. When I asked her what was wrong, she grabbed hold of me and sobbed into my neck. Once I was able to extract myself, I prepared her a cup of hot water (tea, she was very fond of explaining, is somehow bad for your lungs) and I fired up Google Translate to find out exactly what was going on. In a nutshell, she had received a letter from a solicitor in Poland. Her long-estranged husband was demanding a divorce. The part that made her cry was that he also intended to take sole possession of their flat. Wanda couldn't afford a solicitor to contest what was essentially theft, nor could she afford the plane tickets to fly home and resolve it. Basically, in the absence of some sort of intervention from a kind-hearted superhero, she was going to lose her only asset.

Time to put my problem-solving skills to work once again. This particular problem needed money. I didn't have much of it, but I had more than Wanda. When you have no money at all, every problem can feel utterly insurmountable. So, again, as Christ himself would have done, had he just been paid twelve hundred pounds for rewriting the brochure for a knitting supplies company,* I did the decent thing and offered to pay for her plane tickets. I also asked her to think of someone else who might be able to help with the solicitor's fee. There must be someone else? Someone who wasn't me? She shook her head sadly. I gritted my teeth. But I knew that if J was there, he would have told me to stump up for the lot, so after an enormous heartfelt sigh, I offered to pay for that as well. Wanda burst into tears of happiness and wept some more of them into the collar of my t-shirt.

I imagined J's proud face as I told him – he'd tip me a wink and tell me what an old softie I was. As it happens, J would have actually restricted his kindness to the plane tickets, and I was in a not immoderate amount of trouble for writing a blank cheque to a Polish legal firm when the money was earmarked for the bathroom J was designing. (J had, for some utterly unknowable reason, taken over as project manager in our new flat.)

We then had a nice long argument – a month to be precise, because that's how long Wanda was in Poland. When she returned, she threw her arms around us, awash with joy and gratitude. With our help, she'd more than matched her husband's legal firepower and they'd reached a satisfactory settlement. Also very importantly, she'd stood up to the man

---

* 'Needle little help choosing something? We've got some purls of wisdom!' Hey, it's a living.

who expected her to just lay down and do nothing, and she wouldn't have been able to do it without us. Before I could even open my mouth or take the smallest of bows, J replied that it was nothing, really. It was everything I could do not to rat him out – 'You wouldn't have got anything if it wasn't for me!' – but I didn't want to sour the mood, so internalised it into IBS.

Meanwhile, it was fascinating to see another side to Wanda. Compelled perhaps by a genuine sense of gratitude, she was actually being nice to me. It was disconcerting, like if you found out that Skeletor spent his weekends volunteering at a food bank. Then she saw the state of the living room, declared that we were disgusting, filthy animals and that our new cushions were horrible and would have to go. Life returned to normal.

Wanda continued to fuck around with our flat, fiddling with a few things every week, never totally satisfied with their whereabouts. Or even their existence. J would sometimes have to text her to ask where she'd moved all the mugs (under the sink) or all our tote bags (in the bin – 'What is this? Bag museum?'). One day, she'd rearranged the pieces on the chess board so they were in a single block in the middle of the board, alternating black and white. She once threw away a shirt that I'd had dry cleaned because she didn't want the chemicals to give her cancer – then smoked another cigarette. One thing she would never throw away though was food, even when visibly pestilent, and occasionally she'd gather up all the fruit we had and boil it on the hob along with various savoury spices to make litres and litres of some kind of purulent paste, half of which she'd take home in one of our Tupperware containers that we would never see again. The rest she would leave for us to throw away in our own time.

One day, J and I came home together to find Wanda mopping the kitchen in floods of tears. We pretended not to notice and fled to the bedroom to regroup. As if deciding how to best dismember the person we'd accidentally killed, we had a panicked argument about whose turn it was to speak to her (mine again, of course) and what kind of budget we had to resolve it. But this time money couldn't help. Wanda's ex-husband had taken his own life. She should never have gone to Poland, she said. She should never have fought him. She should have just let him have the flat. He needed it more than her. He couldn't live without it. I told her this was the grief talking and that it was probably nothing to do with her going to Poland or fighting him over the flat – nothing to do with anything in any way connected to my funding of her trip, which now felt perilously close to blood money.

There are a million reasons why people kill themselves, I told her. It was probably a combination of many different things. 'Oh, what do you know?' she snapped, lashing out from the cruel shell of her grief.

'Well', I reminded her, 'I am a doctor.'

'Of genitals!' she sobbed.

I made her a mug of hot water and her crying eventually burned out. I told her to go home and take as much time off as she needed. Not extreme amounts but, you know, whatever. She gathered up her stuff and we hugged at the front door. I said I was deeply sorry if I'd somehow contributed to the situation. 'Of course you did,' she said.

My communication skills training, such as it was, hadn't geared me up for being accused of murder. I stuttered slightly.

'Never on purpose, ah?' she said, then smiled. 'You don't like stupid joke?'

– FLASHBACK –

Communication Skills

Ever since doctors wore top hats and footlong beards and prescribed people cocaine or 'a wank',* medical school training has consisted of lectures, tutorials and cutting open dead bodies, leading up to a couple of years of traipsing round hospital wards trying to learn our glutei† from our antecubital fossae.‡ In an effort to acknowledge the new millennium, my medical school hacked back on the lectures,§ chucked us onto the wards a bit earlier and introduced a brand new module for my cohort to contend with: communication skills.

---

* Some urologists still recommend regular ejaculation in the management of chronic prostatitis.

† Arses.

‡ Elbows.

§ It was extremely rare to get anything like a full house in a medical school lecture. Standing room only, though, was a session run by some A&E consultants on terror medicine: what our roles would be as medical students in the case of a terrorist atrocity or other large-scale emergency. This obviously felt vital – god forbid, if such an event happened and we were called upon, we needed to be at the top of our game. We hypothesised among ourselves the potential heroics we'd be expected to perform. The lights dimmed. 'In the event of a major incident, all medical students must congregate in the postgraduate education centre foyer, where you will each be asked to donate a unit of blood.' Oh.

When you think about the best way to learn how to communicate, you might imagine collaborative workshops, interactive brainstorming sessions and teaming up to solve real problems you'll encounter on the wards. Guess again. That's all far too woolly and touchy-feely for a profession whose idea of compassionate leave is to send you to the break room for five minutes to 'calm down'. Medical schools taught communication via ritual humiliation, inspired by TV cop show interrogations.

One student would sit in a windowless room, delivering the kind of general doctorly patter they'd one day find themselves doling out, but with an actor playing the part of a patient or relative. To further compound the anxiety and awkwardness of this am-dram production of *Holby City*, a wall-mounted camera filmed every awkward stutter and silence, broadcasting it live to the room next door, where the rest of the group and the tutor would sit, laughing, judging and supposedly making notes.

I was up first. Student Zero. My task was to tell a relative that his mother had suffered a stroke and was unlikely to make it through the night. I walked into the room to find my actor in floods of frankly hysterical tears. There's little worse than a middle-aged man hamming it up in a workplace role play. His dreams of the National long dead, he'd devoted his career to making life difficult for a bunch of terror-stricken medical students. It was fine though. I had this.

I sat opposite him, introduced myself and tried to keep control of my voice, which sounded like I was driving over cobbles in a 2CV. I explained that his mother – very sadly – had suffered a stroke and as a result, was terribly unwell. Indeed, she was so unwell that if her condition were to deteriorate, which seemed likely, then she would – most probably and also very sadly, and very soon thereafter – become dead. The wailing and gnashing of teeth intensified. *Alright, Dame Judi, rein it in.* He asked what we were doing to keep her alive, which, considering I'd been training to be a doctor for less than a week, felt slightly unfair, so I kept it vague.

'We've been giving her some medicines,' I said, 'and some . . . oxygen?'

He seemed satisfied with this and asked if there was anything else we could do. I suggested – and this was possibly where it all went awry – that we might be able to do an operation.

He was on this in a flash. 'What kind of operation?' he wanted to know. Well, of course he did. We both did. 'Doctor?' he asked, with a flinty glint in his eye, curious as to what kind of hitherto unmentioned surgical intervention could pull his beloved mother back from the very mandibles of death. At this point, knowing how many people were watching on CCTV, I should have said, 'Sorry, Sir, I really don't know what I'm talking about. If you wait here, I'll go and find someone with more than absolutely zero experience.'

Instead, undiluted panic sent my bullshit gland into overdrive and I announced that we would operate . . . on her heart. The actor saw this as his opportunity to play with me, like a panther pawing at a duckling.* He wiped the tears from his eyes and took his time, imagining the chill of a gold-plated Oscar against his skin. Then he asked, 'Sorry, doctor. What exactly *is* a stroke?'

---

* I was too exhausted from the wolf-panini email chain to get into a debate about this one.

Son of a bitch. I paused. I should know this one – doctoring was in my blood. Besides, it felt like the question you answer to win a hundred quid in the perfunctory first round of *Who Wants to be a Millionaire?* Eventually, I told him that it was a type of . . . heart . . . attack?* I heard shrieking laughter on the other side of the stud wall, which I took to be a bad sign.

My waterboarding over, I headed next door for feedback. My tutor replayed the tape. I still find it excruciating to see myself on video: the way the camera adds eight stone, the campness of my voice that I never hear when I'm speaking ('Ooooh! A heart attack!'), the fact I never know what to do with my hands. This was even more excruciating than ever, thanks to the roaring laughter of my peers. All I could focus on were my eyes: pleading with the actor to take it easy on me, not to expose me for the fraud I knew I was.

'Let's start by talking about things that we think went well,' said the tutor.

'Well, he got his name right.'

'He was facing the right way.'

'He spoke English. I think?'

All that was missing was a set of stocks and some angry villagers with rotten cabbages. I didn't want them to see my face: I wasn't going to cry, I just couldn't face the weight of their stares. So I looked at my feet.

I suppose it was character building. But you can say that

---

* I might not have been able to describe a stroke as a lack of blood flow to the brain caused either by a blockage in a blood vessel or an area of haemorrhage, but I could at least have hashed something together using the phrase 'medically floppy' and that thing about smelling toast.

about anything, from a headmaster's beating to a ten-year hostage situation. It doesn't make it right.*

At the end of the lesson, we were each handed our VHS tape to bring back every week to have each subsequent session recorded onto, so we could follow our improvement over the year. I'm not sure how much better I got at communicating with patients but I got a lot better at the feedback sessions afterwards. I realised that my colleagues' criticism came from a place of fear, to distract from the fact they weren't up to the task either. You can learn biochemical pathways and the composition of gallstones all you want – telling someone that their mum's dying is never not awful.

I learned to laugh along, to make a joke of myself and never let them see how I felt inside, never exposing my vulnerability. And when it was their turn, I let them have it in return. Up went the shields, and it would be a long time before they came down again.

---

* I'd reap the benefits in years to come – no one-star book review could ever come close to this kind of flensing.

Chapter 12

A day full of ghosts. The first spectre at my feast came in the shape of an email from my mother with 'Wasn't he in your year at school?' and a link to a piece in the *Telegraph*. I flicked through the article. Yes, he was in my year at school – you know that because he came to our house about three hundred times and you remain good friends with his parents. How nice to see that he's now a high-flying professor of medical genetics. What could the subtext possibly be, mother? I reply with 'I don't remember.' I had stupidly assumed that as time drifted on, she'd realise the odds of me going back to medicine were lower than Charles and Di getting back together. Maybe she'll never stop, even when she has to communicate with me via a medium on *Most Haunted*.

And then a text from my friend Nick. 'Have you heard the news about Bucky?' I hadn't. I had barely even thought about Bucky since we all worked together as obstetric SHOs. 'What's happened?' No reply. Although, given Nick was now a labour ward consultant, it was possible he had something more pressing to do than respond to my texts.

Bucky was never going to stay in obs and gynae. In fact, he spent the entire year I knew him plotting his way out and making sure his payslips would be considerably more impressive as a result. Generally speaking, doctors aren't in it for the money – there are much easier ways to turn a slew of excellent A levels into cold hard cash. Working in the City, for instance. Even a middle-management role at Millets pays better (and – I've never sold someone a mid-price tent, so I'm guessing here – involves far less emotional trauma). But like the generalisation that doctors tend not to murder their patients, there is always the odd exception. Bucky's masterplan was to switch to general practice, set up a private clinic and specialise in vanity: the disease of the rich.

He had it all mapped out and would often excitedly expound on the amounts you could charge for some quasi-medical treat-ment for a drooping face. Such ambitions are supposed to be frowned upon but I was always secretly jealous that he had a gameplan. After a demoralising, blood-splattered, overrunning shift, I was staring down a future full of thousands more de-moralising, blood-splattered, overrunning shifts; Bucky was counting them down like dates on a prison calendar before he could skip off towards millionaire's row. People talk about 'jumping off the treadmill' but when a treadmill moves as fast as medicine, it's remarkably difficult. Have you ever tried jumping off a treadmill at ten miles an hour? You'd break both your legs.

I looked him up on Facebook. Turns out, his plan worked. He'd made it! And also: he'd gone fucking bananas!

Here is a list of life moments he chose to share (presumably proudly): Bucky checking into the Ritz; a photo of Bucky's new Louis Vuitton shoes; Bucky being accepted into some exclusive polo club; Bucky joining UKIP; Bucky drinking cocktails in Dubai while inexplicably dressed as a racing driver; Bucky boasting of evenings spent at the Playboy Club; a video about why anti-depressants don't work; Bucky posing next to a car that was wildly more expensive than my flat; an inspirational quote by Vladimir Putin; Bucky at the Savoy; a 9/11 truther video with a comment from Bucky about the 'emergence of a geo-political New World Order domination'; Bucky back at the Ritz. His strange and well-travelled braggadocio was all funded by his new career as a self-described anti-ageing specialist and expert in cellular degradation, whatever the fuck that may be.★

That evening, Nick texted me a link to a GMC hearing. Long words, yada yada, long words. I skipped to the outcome: immediate erasure from the medical register. Crikey. As every sagging buttock held up by an injection of cow placenta eventually finds out, all good things must come to an end.

Bucky's end was care of a Sunday Times journalist who turned up at his clinic with an athlete, a hidden camera and the question, 'Can you prescribe us some performance-enhancing drugs?' With one hand on his prescription pad and the other extended outward for the thwack of a stuffed brown envelope, Bucky gave a big fat yes and, for good measure, boasted about another hundred or so athletes he'd previously performance-enhanced. Despite Bucky tweeting emphatically that he'd done nothing wrong, the GMC thought they should bring him in for a little chat. In a classic of the 'You can't fire me – I quit!' genre, Bucky emailed the GMC to inform them he'd left the country. The GMC then pointed out that it didn't really work like that and struck him off anyway.

I send the link onto my mum. 'See, I'm not the only person in my year who left medicine!'

★ The desire to look young is a puzzling one, particularly because it's something that can never be achieved. The best you can hope for is a Crimestoppers photofit approximation of youth – a frozen forehead, puffed-up yet strangely solid lips and a stunted ski-jump nose.

Chapter 13

'Have you written anything I might have seen?' asked half the guests at the wedding. Probably not. The first few years of any writer's credits look like the senseless pukings of a random TV show generator: two episodes of a Canadian daytime soap, then script editing a sitcom; six months writing sports reports, then an episode of *Teletubbies*. It's a numbers game: you apply for every job under the sun and a percentage will come good. The guests would give me a pitying wince and then say, 'Oh, you should write for *Doctor Who*!' Sure, yeah, I'll email them now.

This being a family wedding, I was also surrounded by doctors, who provided their own variety of pity. Some treated me like a leper★ and others wondered if I was 'going back'. Are people who worked in a sandwich shop over their school holidays constantly harangued by the bread community about returning to a life of buttering wholemeal? Even if I wanted to, it was out of my hands − I'd just received a letter from

---

★ That's not quite fair − they would have been interested in a leper. One of the drugs used to treat leprosy, rifampicin, has the exciting side effect that it makes all your bodily excretions turn brown, so I'd have been surrounded by doctors eager to see me squeeze out a poo-coloured tear.

the GMC informing me that because I hadn't seen a patient in so long, they were taking away my licence. I kept this to myself though, in case it got back to my mother and ruined the occasion.

I always thought I looked good in a tux, so it was a bit of a blow to be wearing my best suit and for J to announce that I looked absolutely terrible. To be fair on him, I didn't feel that great either – hot, sweaty and generally knackered. I'd put it down to a combination of arguing with relatives, the Gobi-level temperatures and rather too much 'well, it is a wedding after all' every time a bottle of prosecco came within a 200-metre radius of my flute.

Then, in a barefaced attempt to upstage the bride, I fainted. Luckily, a number of the dozen or so doctors eating canapés around me were ready to jump in and start tutting and telling me to pull myself together. The general feeling was that my high pulse and temperature probably meant I had an infection somewhere and it would be a good idea to get some antibiotics on board ASAP. Unfortunately, the only antibiotics at the wedding were in my mother's handbag and were reserved for an emergency, in which category my brief sally into unconsciousness apparently did not fall.

Much as I don't like seeing doctors, I didn't have the strength to protest the next morning. J recounted the story of my funny turn to a nurse in the hospital. He went full Brontë – how I turned 'white as a bedsheet', my 'thready, diaphanous pulse'. I waded in to say he was being melodramatic, but then I started wheezing quite badly and couldn't finish my sentence, which didn't necessarily help my argument.

Stethoscopes, blood tests and X-rays pointed towards pneumonia and a couple of weeks of antibiotics. After all this, when my breathing still sounded like a milk frother, they organised an echocardiogram to take a look at my heart. If you ever have your heart imaged, you very much hope that the report says, 'Absolutely tip top – are you sure your date of birth is correct? You've got the ticker of a twenty-year-old.' What you don't want are sharp intakes of breath and dark, mumbling concerns about how some bits are too thick and other bits are too thin.

Baffled as to why my heart was quite as crap as it was, they flailed around for explanations. Had I had a childhood infection that involved my valves? Was I absolutely certain I hadn't had a heart attack in the past? With my hand on my slightly moth-eaten heart, I told them I was certain. What I didn't tell them, and in retrospect probably should have, was that as a medical student, for the best part of a year, I was in a permanent state of starvation. Stupidly, ridiculously, my embarrassment overruled my ability to let the people who wanted to help me actually help me.

Patients often forget to tell their doctors things. I was just being forgetful.

– FLASHBACK –

Starvation

Feedback has come a long way from 'How's my driving?' stickers on the back of vans. I wouldn't dream of booking a restaurant or a holiday without first spending many thankless hours combing through ten years of nanoquibbles on TripAdvisor. Any online purchase larger than a cable tie is preceded by a systematic appraisal of every single rating it has ever received. And if I'm feeling miserable, I head on over to Amazon and check out the one-star reviews of books by people I hate.

But it's not all about positive things like consumer confidence and revelling in the fact that hundreds of readers agree with me about the wellness charlatan who slagged off my suit at those book awards: sometimes feedback can radically affect your life. For me, it came from the fourth person I ever slept with. In my third year at medical school, after an afterparty for some tedious inter-university rowing race, I found myself back at the flat of a student from another med school. He had seen through my wafer-thin hetero-alpha demeanour and propositioned me at the bar. I had seen through the lycra he was wearing and immediately agreed. I'll spare you a cox joke.*

I assumed from his confidence that he had a lot more miles on the fuckometer than me, so naturally, and using skills I would perfect in my subsequent decade on the hospital wards, I pretended to be a lot more experienced and competent than I actually was. After putting on my bedroom A-game for what I might as well claim was three hours because it's my book and you can't prove otherwise, we were lying in a sweaty post-coital tessellation when he told me, with lethal indifference, that my performance was 'pretty good for a big lad'.

I thanked him because I'm British, then slowly, silently began to digest and deconstruct this perfect example of the backhanded compliment. It meant nothing, I knew that – he meant nothing. It was just a mindless six-word neg, a meaningless joke. And yet . . . it burrowed into my brain and bones like a tumour.

It hadn't previously occurred to me that I might be a big lad. I'd always thought I was just a . . . normal-sized lad? In reality, of course, I was an entirely normal-sized lad. I'd give my left leg to weigh that amount today – in fact I'd *have* to give my left leg to weigh that amount today, plus my right leg and a couple of forearms. But this bloke said I was a big lad, so that's what I was. Bagged and tagged, like a corpse fished out the river.

I know my exact weight that day because I weighed myself and wrote it in my diary the moment I got home. I then weighed myself and documented it between two and eight times a day for the next year. It became clear

----

* I didn't though, did I? I had my cox and ate it.

to me that something had to be done and that a normal diet wasn't going to cut either the mustard (3.5 calories per teaspoon) or my thick layer of adipose tissue. I needed to lose weight much faster than ordinary diets could promise, otherwise the notches on my bedpost were clearly going to top out at four, save perhaps for the odd pity fuck or big-lad fetishist.

So I stopped eating. I initially stopped eating entirely, for five days. It would have been longer, but the ravenously hungry part of my brain eventually overruled the self-destructive, self-conscious part of my brain, whereupon I cracked and made myself a cheese sandwich. Followed immediately by half a loaf of sliced white bread, an extra-large Dominos pizza with one separate dip per slice and a tub of ice cream. Immediately I felt better. Then, a short while later, I felt much, much worse.

That was the night I tried out bulimia. It had to happen – every mouthful of the boulder of carbohydrates I'd just consumed negated my week's excellent work, and vomiting seemed like the digestive system's very own version of Ctrl+Z.

I went up to the bathroom, ran a tap to disguise the sounds, then I did it. It all happened in slow motion. Stare down into toilet bowl. Shift weight slightly from knee to knee. Stare down at hand, and extend index finger. Add another digit just to really make it a party and . . . down the throat they went. Nothing. My gag reflex was basically shot – presumably one of the reasons I was, despite my dimensions, 'pretty good'. Off to the kitchen then, to brew myself a delicious mug of warm salt water, then back to the bathroom to neck it.

I regretted my decision the second the tepid brine hit my stomach lining. I wanted desperately to take it back, but the deed was done and my stomach began to churn and lurch, like a cement mixer gone berserk. Hunched over the toilet, my body jerking like a breakdancer hooked up to the mains, the racket from my heaving and groaning was far louder than the sound of the running tap. I can't imagine many foodstuffs regurgitate as poorly as dough. I guess it's designed to stick together come what may and give the pizza topping safe passage. The white bread, pizza crust, cheese and dipping sauce had congealed into a dense bowling ball in my stomach, and its journey back up was like trying to force a brick through a hosepipe. The delivery was going excruciatingly badly, with no forceps on standby.

After what felt like a full nine months, my oesophagus finally succeeded in squeezing up a bolus of greasy concrete. It was somewhere between a golf ball and a tennis ball, like a beef tomato or a toddler's fist. As soon as it hit the back of my throat, I choked and involuntarily clamped my mouth shut on it, so the dough, with nowhere left to go, squeezed its way up into my nose and its associated maze of sinuses. Not only was this acutely painful, it didn't feel ideal medically, blocking passages that are more traditionally used for the free flow of oxygen. Worse still, no amount of sniffing, snorting or swallowing would get the fucking thing to move. Eventually – and with apologies that you have to read this, please know it was worse still for me – I found myself alone in my bedroom with a chopstick. By pushing the chopstick up into alternate nostrils, I was able to force back the doughberg and create small acidic pellets of regurgitated beige that would then drop back down my gullet to safety. Perhaps understandably, I would never attempt anything quite like that ever again. But I wasn't done yet. Medicine is often about looking beyond the obvious to find a bespoke solution to a problem and this was no different, except perhaps for the fact that this was the opposite of medicine: I was attempting to destroy myself.

I wonder what might have stopped me at this point. A random person telling me I looked great? A flatmate overhearing my toilet concerto and asking if I was OK? Stacey Dooley making a documentary about me?

Doctors have it drilled into them that to become ill in any way is inconvenient – 'Who's going to cover your shifts?' 'Are you sure you can't do a caesarean with a broken leg?' 'You've mostly stopped bleeding.' But however much of a burden you're made to feel, nobody would specifically judge you for getting cancer or breaking your collarbone. Mental illness in patients is treated (after a fashion) but when it occurs within medicine's own ranks, there's still a distinctly Victorian attitude – it's seen as either a failing or self-inflicted. You could argue – and I'm sure people would have – that I was the person sticking my finger down my throat, so all I had to do was . . . not? Medics are supposed to be level-headed, infallible and only go weird under the influence of off-duty claret. I may as well have taped MAD CUNT to my forehead and dressed as the Riddler. In the absence of speaking to anyone, it was up to me and me alone to sort this out. The solution I came up with was not as original as I'd imagined it was at the time.

Nowadays it's a recognised compensatory behaviour, a

well-documented attempt to undo the act of eating and its associated feelings of guilt and shame. Back then, I felt certain I was ploughing special new furrows. My masterplan was to take a mouthful of food – biscuits, nuts, chocolate, whatever – then chew it until I'd sucked all the flavour and goodness from it, before spitting it out. Another mouthful, another chew, another spit. All the delicious enjoyment of food, none of the disgusting calories. Obviously, this was not the kind of thing I could do in public, or even in the communal areas of my shared flat. So eating became something that only happened in private – either in toilet cubicles or, more usually, in the privacy of my own bedroom.

At home, crisps and sweets were easiest because I could empty the packet onto my desk before returning the contents to the bag in three or four disgusting gobfuls. Everything else involved spitting into kitchen roll then balling it up and tossing it into the wastepaper bin in my bedroom, which I did, hundreds of times a day. Every few days, I would purchase more kitchen roll and most nights, when everyone else was sleeping, I would empty the day's collection into the big black bin outside. After a week or so of this faff, I bought my own big black bin, which would stay in my bedroom, and which I'd only have to empty every ten days or so. Obviously this meant that my bedroom was a no-go-area as far as guests were concerned. This wasn't an issue: absolutely nobody was coming round. Within the space of a few weeks, I'd gone from a relatively normal young man who enjoyed the occasional casual lycra-clad bonk at a rowing jamboree to a wildly irrational, body-dysmorphic 'big lad', sharing his room with a collection of half-chewed junk food.

The problem was – it was working. Just as I might be entertaining the idea that there could be something wrong with me, someone would tell me how well I looked ('well' of course being code for 'thin') and any doubts I was having would pop like dying bubbles of logic. If I looked remarkably well – well enough to be remarked upon – then how on earth could I possibly be ill?

I'd lost roughly the weight of a toddler by now. Of course, there was no 'roughly' about it, I was keeping obsessive tabs and knew the magic number to within a quarter of a pound, thanks to my freshly purchased set of precision scales, accurate enough for any molecular biologist. I'd actually bought two sets of these scales so I could weigh myself on both and log the more gratifying of the results.

The gamification offered by the scales drove me to further distraction: a few ounces lost meant victory, vindication and knowing that what I was doing was worthwhile. A few ounces gained meant defeat, degradation and the sense that what I was doing was utterly pointless. On bad days, I'd spend hours either running or on the loo, trying to jog or shit myself back into my own good books. I was following a flowchart where every single path led me to behaviour that was increasingly abnormal. I cancelled so many dinners that I eventually confected a gastrointestinal condition – one that was pending investigation and rendered meals all but impossible. Openly telling someone about an issue with mucus in my bowels was a much more comfortable prospect than having anyone suspect I might have an abnormal relationship with food.

I took down the wavy IKEA mirror from my bedroom wall. Like the French author Guy de Maupassant who wrote inside the Eiffel Tower because it was the only place in Paris he couldn't see it, I could just about cope with my body as long as I never caught its reflection.

On it went. Doubt, reassurance, shame, success, failure – a bad day would be followed by a jackpot: another unwitting enabler making the mistake of telling me how well I was looking. Down another jeans size! By now I'd stopped buying kitchen roll and was just spitting food directly into the bin in my bedroom. If I got a headache, I would forsake the paracetamol because . . . well, those calories were avoidable. Yet another pair of jeans! And how well I was looking! Except of course, I wasn't. I looked bloody awful, like I had radiation sickness. A simple equation meant that in the absence of fuel, I had no energy. After a day of lectures I couldn't focus on, I'd be tired enough to sleep for maybe fourteen hours at a stretch. My body would shut down like a laptop. But even this seemed like a good thing: fourteen hours asleep was fourteen hours without food.

My skin was deteriorating – a scaly patina of eczema, something I'd never experienced before, spread from the hollows of my eyes across my brand new cheekbones. My lips were so red and chapped that it looked like I was holding them together with Chanel Rouge. Oh, and my nails were coming off. I was basically Jeff Goldblum in *The Fly*, if Jeff Goldblum were suffering from a catastrophic nutrient deficiency due to self-starvation rather than turning into an arthropod. There was now no way I could be considered a big lad by potential suitors, although that was fairly academic because I hadn't managed anything approaching an erection for weeks. Still, I'd probably be fine. As far as I was concerned, this wasn't an eating disorder – it was just a hobby, really, this thing I did. Besides, like every single one of the billions of addicts before me, I was convinced I could stop at any moment – I just . . . didn't want to, not yet.

Eventually and inevitably, the comments changed. For every person telling me how well I looked, there was another who recoiled slightly, enquired with concern after my health or made a typical medic bad-taste joke about wasting diseases or Michael Stipe. This was the wake-up call I needed. Not about my behaviour, but about a number of toxic friendships I'd clearly been enduring for far too long – I couldn't afford to have jealous, spiteful people like that in my orbit. Meantime, I started wearing baggier clothes, just to keep a lid on the down-talking. Luckily, I already had a wardrobe full of baggy clothes.

I was, in short, a mess. Never previously in danger of winning the 'Most Gregarious Student' rosette, I had moved to another level of solitude: avoiding close to all human contact, cut off from my small circle of friends. I'd successfully extricated myself from all of my commitments, bar one: the annual Music Society weekend away. Three days of constant communal eating and drinking, plus the occasional honk into a trombone. There was no way to get through it without having to eat food with other people – and if I did that, everything I'd been slaving over for months would be ruined. I'd get onto the coach a haunted weirdo with missing fingernails but I'd come back a born-again big lad, my features encased in a squidgy pillow of fat. There was no question of me going. I told them I was unwell. To be fair, you only had to look at me. None of it would wash with them – who were they going to get to play second trombone at such short notice? Trying to weasel out of it was beginning to raise too many eyebrows, my isolationism making it clear that something was wrong. So I agreed to go.

The countdown was excruciatingly stressful. All the delicious control I'd managed to create around food was about to evaporate. Every morning for two weeks beforehand, I went for a long run, just to buy myself some wiggle room. The calories I burned running would be set against anything I ingested if the worst came to the worst and I absolutely had to swallow something.

In the end, somehow, thanks to sleight of hand at buffets and a combination of hankie-spitting, pocket-filling, and hiding it under cutlery at restaurants, I seemed to get away with it. Pretty much. There was one moment when a dorm-mate spotted the weighing scales I'd taken with me – the very thought of not knowing my weight for three days under such trying circumstances was enough to bring on a panic attack.

There was a slight pause when he asked me why I had them, before I said, 'Luggage. I always carry a set of scales with me so that I can weigh my luggage before I leave for the airport. Must still be in there from when I last flew somewhere. Lanzarote – that was it.' He bought my cover story with an uninterested shrug. Thinking about it now, it would have crumbled under the slightest scrutiny.* But convincing or not, I lied more about food in those nine months than I'd cumulatively lied in my whole life ever before. And I kept getting away with it! I must have been fucking good.

I wasn't. When I got back to the flat after the weekend away, Groot was waiting for me by the front door. He was wondering if we could just have a little chat. His tone of voice alone made clear that this was more than a cleaning rota infraction. In my absence, Groot had had to reset the router in my bedroom and, while he was in there, he saw it: an eighty-litre plastic bin three-quarters full of half-chewed food, studded with packets of crisps and Fruit Pastilles. Tadaaaa!

Things began to fall into place for him. Why I never ate in the kitchen any more, why I hadn't been to the pub in a year and why I'd lost a third of my physical presence. My bedroom door was still open and the aroma of my lifestyle choices filtered out through the flat. Faced with the talisman of my deceit, I felt my life crumble all around me. I must have told my flatmates 200 separate, food-related lies and all of them were exposed at once. The times I was ill with some vague intestinal complaint – worse, the sympathy they'd shown me for it. The times I couldn't eat because I'd grabbed something on my way home or

---

*   'So you brought your scales to the airport?'
    'Yeah.'
    'Where they weigh your luggage for you anyway?'
    'Yeah.'
    'And in your case, a good, what, kilogram of that weight is now scales?'
    'Yeah.'
    'Cool . . .'

because I was fasting before my impending colonoscopy or one of that year's multiple Yom Kippurs.

Now the chewed-up Wotsits were out of the bag. They knew for sure: I was a fucking loon. I might have tried to convince myself that my behaviour was harmless, just symptomatic of a more creative approach to life – but there's nothing like thirty kilos of fetid gob-mush to bring you down to earth. I was bang to rights. Policemen must constantly experience the desperate flailing of the totally guilty – swag over their shoulder, blood under their fingernails, yet still they flail. As did I.

'How dare you go into my room!' I thundered. Followed by an abject denial of any knowledge of the bin. Followed by a more pathetic 'You couldn't possibly understand.' And finally begging him not to tell anyone what he'd seen. He promised his silence on the condition that I got the help I needed. I gave him my word. My word was my bond. My bond, however, was nothing – a cardboard sword in a zombie apocalypse; a panini up against a wolf.

Of course I didn't get any help, I was a medic. If I spoke to anyone about it, they'd probably feel obliged to break their duty of confidentiality and alert the Dean of the medical school, the GMC and the Secretary of State for Health, like if I'd confessed to a sudden and uncontrollable taste for human flesh. Even Mike Schachter, who had gently enquired after my health when he'd spotted what was left of me leaving a lecture theatre, might have somehow turned on me. Of course he wouldn't have. And yet . . . what if he did? It wasn't worth the risk.

But I did stop – at least for a while. Much as it began with other people's opinions of me, so other people's opinions of me ended it. Even though I was still in denial about the seriousness of it all, the fear of public exposure far outweighed whatever neuroses were driving me to do it in the first place.

Truthfully, I didn't think I needed to speak to anyone. In my head, I wasn't a particularly serious or interesting case. Even though I'd lost a lot of weight, I'd barely grazed the 'underweight' section of the BMI chart. I hadn't been admitted to hospital and the only tube I'd been fed through said Smarties on the side. Talking about it felt almost fraudulent. After all, what had I done, really? I'd lost some weight. And wasn't losing weight a good thing? Hadn't I learned in my cardiology lectures that fat leads to strokes and heart attacks and all sorts of clogged-up blood vessels? Isn't that why GPs tell at least half their patients that losing a bit of weight wouldn't do them any harm? I'd certainly said the same thing to absolutely droves of patients. I worked in a gynaecology endocrine clinic every Tuesday morning for a year, helping women with poly-cystic ovarian syndrome (PCOS). A large number of the consultations involved a chat about how weight loss might improve their symptoms.

'I've tried everything,' they would often say.

Not quite everything, I would think.

One clinic, a dickwad of a consultant prodded me in the stomach and asked me if I was developing a bit of PCOS myself. I laughed, then spat into the bin for a fortnight, no harm done.

When a journalist called me 'chubby' in a review of a show at the Edinburgh Festival it was a nifty shortcut to losing a bit of weight, no harm done. When someone on Twitter messaged me to say I'd 'piled on the pounds' – a couple of packs of kitchen roll, a few cancelled dinners, no harm done. I never felt cross about the comments either. Rather, I was grateful they'd let me know that I needed to get back on the programme. Fat again, thin again, fat again, thin again.★

I don't blame 'big lad' for starting this off. Obviously. He couldn't know he was unleashing an avalanche of aberrant behaviour. And if it hadn't been him, then it would have been some other trigger at some other point. So I bear him no ill will. I do think about him occasionally, though, and while revisiting this episode, I couldn't resist a little google, just to see what he's up to. According to his hospital's website, he's now a consultant psychiatrist specialising in, among other things, treatment of addiction and eating disorders. I wish his patients the best of luck.

★ I had a brief flirtation with a drug called Orlistat, which works by fucking with an enzyme called lipase. Lipase's day job is to hang around in your small intestine looking for any fat that you've just eaten, break it down into bite-sized molecules that your body can absorb and then store any excess in your waistline. No lipase means no fat absorption means no fat deposits. I ordered myself a crate of it on the internet (anonymously, obviously).

I was out at dinner and ordered French onion soup topped with enough cheese for a decent-sized fondue, followed by an Orlistat chaser to mop up all the horrible fat. I hadn't entirely thought through the physics of it – the cheese still had to go somewhere and, in the absence of being absorbed in the traditional way, it continued heading south, using my gastrointestinal tract like a water flume. The medical term is 'faecal urgency'. Urgency doesn't quite cover it. Faecal panic might be closer. Followed by faecal horror, as I ran to the bathroom while 300g of emulsified cheddar slurped down my leg via my jibbering rectum.

Chapter 14

Whether you call it doing my time at the coalface, an alignment of the stars or a long-overdue recognition of my unmistakeable genius, there had been a definite shift in my writing career. I was assisted down the birth canal of success by taking a shoebox full of my diaries to Scotland and reading them out at the Edinburgh Fringe, the birthplace (and sometimes crematorium) of many a comedian's career. It was basically a live audiobook, except you couldn't skip the boring bits.

One day, there happened to be a publisher in the audience who stayed awake throughout and liked what they heard enough that they offered me a deal to release those diaries as a book. As news of this publishing contract emerged, people started to become more interested in me – mild success often breeds mild success. I certainly wasn't in danger of becoming the next Russell T Davies, but there was now a distinct flow of offers coming in, which meant that I (and presumably Santander) had less of a constant feeling of vomity panic. It also meant I had the luxury of being a little pickier than when I was writing mother-in-law jokes for coked-up best men.

A sample week of email requests from my agent:

Would Adam be interested in writing copy for a campaign about weighted blankets? (No.)

Would Adam be interested in putting himself forward to the producer of a dramatic reconstruction of the 1970s LSD bust Operation Julie? (No.)

We have secured the movie rights to Play-Doh. Would Adam be interested in pitching for this? (No, sounds shitbad.)

Would Adam consider participating in a fundraiser for a dementia charity? (Yes!)

Charity work is always, at least in part, a selfish act – a ten quid pro quo situation. At one end, there's the barefaced version: immortality on a brass plate, behind the velvet curtain you pull open as the cameras flash. Behold the Bannatyne Foundation, the Winfrey Ward, the DiCaprio Donkey Sanctuary. At the other end is the plain old nice warm glow: a feeling that, in a world of eight billion essentially powerless people, you're being of use in some small way. Then, there's that grey area in the middle, loaded with motive and false modesty. The LOOK HOW KIND I AM BUT I REALLY DON'T LIKE TO TALK ABOUT IT social media post.

In my own case, warm glow aside, my willingness to help out with the fight against dementia was prompted by a more pragmatic kind of selfishness, based on the simple fact that of my three grandparents who reached dementable age, 100 per cent of them eventually succumbed. Marble deficit, to some degree or other, was fairly rife in my family. In fact, my last remaining grandparent was deeply mired in dementia at the time of the request. Therefore, assuming I wasn't adopted (and I felt sure by then I'd disappointed my parents enough times that this news would have been blurted out in anger at some point), it made perfect sense for me to do everything in my power to help find a cure now rather than later when, let's face it, I'd probably forget to.

There seem to be two distinct patterns when it comes to dementia: you can either drift off into a seemingly semi-pleasant fog, where everything you've seen or heard or known ebbs painlessly away like melting snow. Or you can be dragged off, kicking and screaming, defiant, terrified and in the worst, most heartbreaking distress you've ever known. Which way you go seems largely determined by how much awareness you have about what's happening to you. And, of course, a horrible cocktail of both options is also available.*

My paternal grandfather's mind plumped primarily for the gentle option, so he drifted away with minimal fuss until he could no longer be cared for in his house and was transferred into a nursing home, albeit one with cushioned vertical surfaces. Every few months, however, his neurons would somehow magically reconnect for a few hours and he'd find himself, for reasons he couldn't possibly understand, horribly alone in a terrifying and unfamiliar prison cell. He'd generally use these windows of lucidity to attempt his escape. On one such occasion, he asked if he might be allowed to take a walk down the high street as a special treat. He dressed himself very smartly in a three-piece suit, as he would always do, and a young male healthcare assistant was assigned to chaperone him, and have him back in his room an hour later.

---

* This analysis is based on personal experience, rather than any kind of actual knowledge. At medical school, you have to take your holiday as annual leave rather than in official term breaks. I took a fortnight of leave in one go, managing to skip the whole of psychiatry and most of neurology in the process.

'Do you mind if I pop in here?' my granddad asked, signalling to a motorcycle showroom midway through his walk. The healthcare assistant nodded and waited by the entrance as my granddad wandered around inside, admiring the dazzling chrome of these machines that he would, in all likelihood, never get this close to again. Then he approached the burly man behind the till and in a perfectly pitched tone of reasonable concern, said something along the lines of, 'I'm very sorry to bother you, but would you mind calling the police? That young man in the doorway has been following me. I'm afraid he might want to harm me in some way.' Unfortunately, though understandably, the shop staff chose to take the word of the well-spoken, smartly dressed elderly gentleman over the acne-scarred, unkempt school leaver in a tracksuit, and while the latter was detained by a couple of retired Hells Angels, my granddad was free to wander the streets of East London for nearly ten hours before he was recaptured.

Although the healthcare assistant only spent a very short while in police custody before his story was verified and a search party dispatched, the nursing home was furious with my parents. They essentially acted like this was some kind of meticulously planned *Ocean's Eleven*-style heist in which the whole family was complicit. In return, my parents were even more furious with the nursing home for their sloppiness.

'You realise he could have *died*?'

But, in a sense, my grandfather already had. Certainly by the time of his physical passing, I'd already done my mourning for the man I knew, who'd kiss the top of your head and berate everything you were wearing, reminding you that, as a former tailor, 'I could make that better myself.'

When you reach your mid-thirties, the chances must be salami-thin that you have any remaining grandparents. I know this because of the surprise that was always expressed when people found out my grandmother was still kicking around. 'And she's sharp as a tack,' I'd always add. Until, of course, she wasn't. Unlike my granddad, whose dementia was, for the most part, a seemingly painless befuddlement, my gran's was a deeply scary, angry time, full of confusion, delusion and hallucination.

'They're back!' she screamed, when I visited her at home for the final time. I asked her who was back. 'The police! They're upstairs.'

'Ah, OK,' I said. 'Let me go check for you.' I nipped upstairs and, like I was looking under the bed for monsters, popped my head into the airing cupboard and the avocado bathroom in search of armed response units.

I couldn't persuade her she wasn't under siege, so I reverted to medical mode – nodding, smiling, asking straight-faced follow-up questions. 'Why do you think there are so many police officers here? What do you think they want?'

Talking about it made her less agitated, so I kept going – it felt like I was helping rather than humouring her. The human brain is quite incredible. Even while malfunctioning so badly that she couldn't remember my name, she was still able to construct a dramatically satisfying narrative about a rota of police officers staking out the spare bedroom to spy on an international drugs ring in the house across the street. I marvelled at her brain's impressive improv – they had names, backstories and bad habits.

I felt more comfortable trying to deal with this as a doctor rather than as a grandchild. A doctor always gets to walk away and not think about it afterwards. But of course I still thought about her – a sickness in the pit of my stomach that she had retreated so far into this nightmare fantasy world. I channelled my inner Vulcan, cauterised my tear ducts and reported back to my parents as if I were a specialist they'd asked to assess the patient. 'She is increasingly thought-disordered, with evidence of visual and auditory hallucinations.' I advised them *a home* would probably be more appropriate at this point than *her home*.

A few weeks after I performed at the dementia benefit show, my grandma had her own final gig. Orthodox Jewish funerals lean needlessly towards the bleak – they're no celebration of life, no New Orleans jazz send-off. Just a morbid, miserable reminder that no matter how we live our lives, we're all simply waiting to feed the worms. Death, like life, is no excuse for a party.

She lay plonked in a plain, unadorned coffin in the middle of a functional, joyless building with the design aesthetic of a recycling centre. There would be no music and no singing. The rules dictated men and women must be segregated and forced to stand on opposite sides of the room, to prevent husbands and wives from consoling each other and escaping any of the necessary, character-building anguish. No heartening hymns, just impenetrable, monotonous Hebrew prayers that I pretended to join in with, mouth opening and shutting like a garage door – a footballer blagging the national anthem.

But Judaism's best efforts were no match for my family's iron resolve, half of whom had also received further training at medical school, and a regional Kleenex shortage was avoided.

This was the first Jewish funeral I'd been to that was in any way pimped up – my grandmother had written her own eulogy and, after some moderate kvetching, the rabbi eventually agreed to read it out.

'I was born in 1926,' he began, unsettlingly, his thick Israeli accent giving the whole thing a definite séance vibe.* Despite the weirdness of it, it was fascinating to hear what Grandma had to say from the other side. There were vast swathes of her life I had no idea about, such as the many years she spent as a foster carer. Then there was the story of how she met my granddad, a meet-cute I would have otherwise never known about. Then there was the time the police staked out her spare bedroom to spy on an international drugs ring in the house across the street. Hang on, what?!

I spent the remaining forty minutes of the service trying to make sense of what I'd just heard. If this police story was *true*, did I unnecessarily expedite her hospital admission by saying she was more demented than she actually was? I must have looked particularly traumatised because J squeezed my hand and flashed me a comforting smile. I batted him away. I'm not sure what god's views on homosexuality are but given the segregation arrangement, it felt like even if this was technically allowed then it really wasn't in the spirit of the law.

Due to a longstanding family rift that even death could not heal,† my corner of the family didn't attend the main wake and instead decamped to a greasy spoon down the road. I ordered an omelette and chips, but then my mum told me that my suit was looking tight on me so I just stared at my plate in silence instead. When I'd got over my funereal fat-shaming, I questioned her about the contents of the auto-eulogy. The police had indeed staked out my grandmother's spare bedroom

---

* J pointed out afterwards that it would have been much better if she'd started with a nice long 'WooOOOOooo!'.

† Were I to disclose it here, it would result in the immediate double-suicide of my parents, so I'm saving that reveal for when I really need it.

but not a few weeks ago as her dementia had claimed, rather, back in the mid-1970s.

The boys in blue bell bottoms had cottoned on to a vast drugs enterprise, based out of a fairly inconspicuous house in Seymour Road, Hampton Wick, directly opposite my grandparents'. And so, day and night for a very long time, a pair of officers took turns camping out in their spare room with a set of binoculars. The cover story was that my grandparents were having building work done, so at every change of shift, a new duo replaced the last pair, all wearing workmen's overalls and carrying identical metal tool-boxes. This apparently raised lots of eyebrows among the curtain twitchers of Seymour Road. What kind of building work, they wondered, went on for months at a time but was utterly silent and resulted in no discernible improvements to the house? Why had this previously sociable couple closed their doors to their neighbours? And – weirdest of all – what kind of silent construction necessitated twenty-four-hour-a-day shiftwork? As far as their neighbours were concerned, there was only one reasonable explanation: they were clearly kinky sex perverts, whose appetite for unthinkable activities was so insatiable that they required a constant supply of young men dressed as builders.*

After a full year of staking out, the police finally had the evidence they needed and decamped from upstairs. Although they never offered any financial compensation to my grandparents for the use of the room, they did cough up a few quid when my grandmother pointed out that the mattress was completely ruined, thanks to an entire year of

---

* In truth, this predilection skipped a couple of generations.

24/7 chain smoking. No doubt when my granddad dumped a stained and knackered mattress in the front garden it did little to dispel the street's working theory. I asked my mum questions till she ran out of answers. 'Oh, look it up!' she eventually cried, exasperated. 'It's called Operation Julie. It's quite famous.'*

Of course Grandma would have housed a famous drugs sting. How could she not? I was slightly ashamed that I hadn't believed she was telling some version of the truth, or at least investigated a little further than checking behind the out-of-date matzos in the kitchen cupboard.

My agent was more than a little surprised by my 180-degree change of heart regarding the Operation Julie project. Not only did I now definitely want to meet the producers but I was certain I was the perfect writer for the job, and had already constructed a detailed B-plot concerning the mild-mannered sting-enablers across the street. Unfortunately, by the time of my turnaround, they'd already found another writer. (Probably Russell T Davies.)

It's just as well – I would have had a thousand questions about what happened and no one to answer them, only the recurring guilt that I never had these discussions with my grandmother while she was alive. What an uneven distribution of interest we had in each other's lives: she followed every aspect of mine, from my birthweight to my postgraduate exam results, and I'd barely thought to ask her anything. There are always uneven

---

* The amateur chemists spilled so much LSD on the carpet, literally dropping acid – no, you can't have a refund on the book – that when the rozzers left my grandparents' spare room and raided the lab, they ended up tripping their faces off. The raid knocked out most of the LSD in the UK, sending the price of the humble acid tab up 500 per cent and causing untold misery in halls of residence and swingers' parties across the country.

relationships in life – one partner not quite feeling it so much; selfish friends who go to ground whenever you have a problem but expect unlimited counselling if they stub a toe – but perhaps the most cruel and unjust of all is the disservice we do to those who've waited all their lives to meet us. What a wretch of a grandson I was. I guess things evened out right at the end though, when she was alternating between calling me my granddad's name, my brother's name and Alvin, whoever the fuck Alvin is.*

There's a clear invisibility to the very elderly, where we fail to see them as people with at least twice our lived existence. We forget, as they dribble onto their misshaped cardigans, drink their hyper-sweetened tea and keep the doily industry going, that they were and are real people. Like the light coming from a long-dead star, they once laughed, sang and kissed strangers; fought, lied and kept secrets. Medicine is often guilty of letting the elderly blend into an amorphous homogeneity – wrinkled bags of skin and warfarin.†

---

* There is a chance, of course, that the Seymour Road Residents' Association was right all along and 'Alvin' was one of dozens of gentlemen callers. This is going to open up another rift within the Kay family, isn't it?

† At one hospital I worked in, there was a rather wonderful idea that above every elderly patient's bed there should be a photograph of them in their youth. On stage at the Coliseum. At the bottom of a ski slope. It was meant to serve as a reminder of their individuality, and a fun conversational amuse-bouche before getting onto the main course of their bedsore management. But at the same time, there was a slight emptiness to it – the idea that hard evidence of their former youth was the only way we could humanise them. Maybe one day geriatric patients will seek validation through recordings of TikTok dances they performed in their twenties. Regardless, the hospital's vintage photo system went to shit after a couple of months, coming to a head when a patient's wife wondered why her elderly husband had a photo of a lithe young woman in swimwear taking pride of place above his bed. She took some convincing to believe this was a real initiative and that they'd just forgotten to take down a previous patient's youthful portrait.

My parents will be next up, as they shuffle into their position as 'final generation', like the Snickers edging a step forward in the vending machine, the void waiting beneath. It was inconceivable that they weren't thinking this at the funeral, behind their blank faces. I decided to properly speak to them and build a stronger bond, one to last after they've gone. I wouldn't even know where to begin with the first thirty years of their eulogies. And if we're all the products of our childhoods, maybe that would give me a glint of the emotions that I knew must be sloshing around inside them somewhere.

The next time I saw my dad, I sat him down and asked him a few questions. What was his childhood like? Did he have any pets? Where did he go on holiday? He stopped me after about three minutes.

'This isn't going in a book, is it?'

Chapter 15

Lunch with my mum in London. *This is Going to Hurt* was lukewarm off the press and had debuted in the Sunday Times bestsellers list. Not at number one, as she didn't hesitate to remind me, but it was there. A mere seven years since I left medicine, she even managed a full meal without asking if I'll need to get my stethoscope serviced before reapplying for a registrar post, or sharing news clippings of heroic doctors. She wasn't quite pointing to me and saying 'My son, the author!' but I could detect a flicker of pride. Sometimes the biggest plaudits come from words not said.

It occurred to me that the reason we never spoke much about my job writing for telly wasn't just the fact it represented my escape from medicine. It simply wasn't her world. She hadn't heard of any of the shows I'd written for (in fairness, nor had 97 per cent of the country) and even if she were to watch them, they really wouldn't have been her cup of camomile. But books! She read books. I mean, she hadn't read *my* book, but she told me she intended to.*

The bill arrived and she said that as I was now a famous author, surely I was able to pick up the tab? I started to spit my excuses and she laughed slightly too hard and got out her credit card. She told me she'd love to see my book in the window of a bookshop – should we wander past one? I'd love to see my book in the window of a bookshop too, pal. I explained that I couldn't promise a window but there was a decent chance we could find one on a shelf somewhere, so we wandered to a slightly swanky bookshop around the corner.

I was killing two birds with one brick, actually: my publisher would have wanted me to pop in. Any time you pass a bookshop, head in! Introduce yourself! Offer to sign any copies they've got! A signed book is a sold book!

Maybe other authors are more shamelessly outgoing than me, but the very thought of wandering into a shop and proclaiming myself the grand originator of something they may or may not actually have in stock makes my anus constrict to a pinhole and my pulse thrash out the drum fill from 'In the Air Tonight'. After announcing myself to a few bookshops who didn't have a copy, I'd learned that the safest procedure for my self-worth was not to introduce myself as an author but to go full JR Hartley and simply make a casual enquiry as an interested punter. 'Do you happen to have any copies of *This is Going to Hurt* by . . . I think it's . . . Adam Kay?' If so, I would then – surprise! – announce myself as the author like I was jumping out of a birthday cake and offer to scribble on them

---

* In my second book, *Twas the Nightshift Before Christmas*, the dedication on the first page reads, 'To my parents'. Followed overleaf with, 'Not really to my parents, but they won't read beyond that page.' My mum phoned me a few days after publication to thank me for the kind dedication. She still hasn't noticed.

with a Sharpie. At this point, they would presumably wonder why I struggled to remember my own name.

We walked in and I scanned the shelves for a copy. Nope. 'There's probably been a run on them,' suggested my mum.

I made my way to the till to have an excruciating conversation. 'Do you happen to have any copies of *This is Going to Hurt*?' The lady behind the till thought they had it out the back and wandered off to check. I was about to do my big reveal to the man still behind the counter when he told me he'd already read it and it wasn't really his thing – he didn't know why it had been bothering the charts. It tries a bit too hard to be funny, he said, and fails entirely on that score.★ And that endless swearing, how very clever. He's all for an unlikeable protagonist, he wanged on, but the author of this book just seemed a little bit *too* much of an arsehole. In short, he concluded, in a field of a thousand medical memoirs, I could do a lot better. Paul Kalanithi's *When Breath Becomes Air*, perhaps? I couldn't face turning around to see my mother's face.

The lady returned shortly with a copy of my book and asked if I'd like to buy it. Yes I fucking would, actually: someone had to defend my book's honour, even if I was now out of pocket from the entire enterprise. I paid (cash – to avoid showing the name on my debit card) and we left.

My mother peeked into the bag as if searching for cola bottles in the pick 'n' mix. 'Do you think I might borrow that?'

★ 'And the footnotes add nothing.'

Chapter 16

My friend Tony's son had died in an accident – an unimaginable cruelty. I sat on my own near the back of the small church and counted the tiles on the floor to shut my ears off from the words being said. I looked at the joinery of the half-sized coffin instead of thinking about the child inside or his poor family. My physical presence was in the church, but nothing more.

I didn't stay for the wake. I couldn't. I told myself they probably just wanted their inner circle there but truthfully, I couldn't face it. Medicine introduced me to a lot of grief but it always allowed me to step away straight afterwards. I knew that I was leaving heartbreak in my slipstream but I never had to fully confront it – there would be something else to fill the space. Usually in obstetrics it was a joyful thing, a new life to cleanse the palate. Sometimes it was another crushing blow. But I could still leave it behind afterwards. Unlike Tony.

'How are you doing?' I asked him as I left the church. What a clumsy, stupid thing to say, as if the answer could be anything other than *absolutely inexpressibly fucking terrible*. 'I'm looking at it like this,' he said. 'The worst possible thing that can ever happen in my life has happened. Assuming I manage to continue, then life can only ever feel better.' What the hell are you meant to say in reply to that? I hugged him awkwardly and he thanked me for coming.

Someone else came up to him and spoke much more eloquently, much more kindly, with all the right words. It sounded like they worked together. Why could some bloke from a trading floor communicate more compassionately than me, who was apparently trained in it? Had I lost my touch or did I never actually have it? Did I make every loved one feel like their loss was just another line on a spreadsheet?

I thought a lot about grief on the train back home. I always dealt in a very strange type: breaking bad news about the baby a family was expecting to meet and now never would. When someone you know dies, your memories become the buffer between you and the abyss, the residual glow of your shared experiences still shining the tiniest particles of light into your darkness. They were here, you were together, and their memory prevails for as long as you're alive to keep it. When an unborn child is taken from you, there is precious little to give you comfort. There are no souvenirs. Every experience you shared was one-sided: moments of hope and excitement, where the future was the only thing that mattered. Grief's usual empty caveats and reassurances don't apply – talk of a good innings, full lives well-lived. There's no book of life to look back through; every page remains blank with expectation, the story ending before anyone was ready.

The train was passing through Warrington when J called to say his sister had given birth. A healthy, bouncing – as people describe them for some reason – baby boy. I disseminated the happy news round my side of the family. It felt strange – the universe operating some one-in-one-out system.

'How nice for her mum,' replied my mother. It felt deeply

loaded, so I asked her what she meant by that. 'It's just nice for her mum – it's very special being a grandmother.'

I didn't have the emotional wherewithal for this chat, not now. 'Look, I don't know why it's not happening for us – it's been years since we used protection.' She tutted and hung up.

– FLASHBACK –

No Souvenirs

H was pregnant, having an ultrasound in the hospital where I worked. I'd been able to ensure she got the absolute best silver service treatment available – a senior consultant, no less, performing the scan. In the waiting room, all the doctors and midwives smiled at me as they walked past. I whispered to H which of them were shit and she laughed; humour my perpetual pin to burst those awkward emotional bubbles, whether at home, at work or here – a weird amalgam of the two.

In the scanning room, I provided a running commentary.

Now he's measuring the length of the leg.

Did you know that before ultrasound gel was invented, people had to be scanned underwater?★

I'm not sure if I was trying to be reassuring, showing off my obstetric onions, or if I was just papering over the

---

★ Ultrasound is descended from Sonar and it took a while to shake off the whole 'transmitting through water' thing: for decades patients had to sit extremely still in a water bath. Ultrasound's first medical application was in fact therapeutic rather than diagnostic, being used to destroy brain tissue in patients with chronic pain. Luckily, they soon worked out how to turn the power down (and it's now entirely safe).

anxiety I felt with whatever medical blather came into my head.

That setting measures the blood flow, you'll hear a swooshing noise in a second – there you go.

He's just zooming in there to have a look at something.

Oh . . . no, nothing, just . . . that doesn't look great actually . . .

And then I collapsed – a proper full-blown, like-they-do-on-the-telly collapse, where you wake up in a different room wearing an oxygen mask, surrounded by people in scrubs yammering medical terminology. In this case, of course, the people in scrubs were my colleagues. Instantly, I felt more humiliated than I think I'd ever been in my life. Not only was I pointlessly draining my hospital's already overstretched resources, I was also a giant, multifaceted failure, and publicly so. I had failed as a husband, unable to comfort my wife in her hour of need. I had failed as a doctor, unable to deal with bad news, and I had failed as a human being, gallivanting in and out of consciousness and stealing the limelight when I should have just . . . coped.

In the days that followed, my colleagues compounded my shame. On my way to perform a caesarean, another registrar joked with me whether I would faint during it. Lost for any other reaction, I laughed along, but dark humour is definitely tougher to stomach when you've just lost a child.

If kinder colleagues asked how I was doing, I would minimise my feelings. 'You know, these things happen.' I didn't tell them that I constantly felt like I'd taken a bowling ball to the stomach, that my brain alternated unpredictably between feeling numb and feeling overwhelmed, that I had these strange lapses of unreality, where I felt disconnected from my body and that I was somehow someone else. I didn't tell anyone that.

I spent a week working up the courage to ask a consultant if I could step out of early pregnancy clinics for a while. 'Sure,' he said. 'Just find someone else to do them.' I didn't find anyone else to do them because I was too embarrassed to explain to my colleagues why I couldn't do them myself. I knew they'd think I was being pathetic. The truth is, I thought I was being pathetic. A colleague had been denied the day off when her boyfriend was admitted to ITU: they weren't married so she didn't qualify for compassionate leave. Heavily pregnant doctors were still expected to do shifts on labour ward, taking skin and muscle samples from stillborn children. How did my second-hand experience possibly constitute a reason? I grew to hate my labour ward shifts, where every day I met dozens of people who got to have babies when I wasn't allowed to. I started to feel jealous and resentful, which isn't the ideal look for a doctor.

I didn't feel as if I could talk about any of this at home, either. As far as I was concerned, H was the person who was actually suffering; I was just the plus one at this party and my feelings weren't particularly relevant. So instead, I focused all my attention on trying, very poorly, to make H feel better.

After stumbling through work for a couple of weeks, I asked my consultant if I could have a bit of time off. The answer wasn't no, it was somehow worse. 'Really?' It encapsulated both the impact my absence would have on an already threadbare rota, as well as surprise that I was still struggling so much with such a relative trifle. I backtracked and said I was actually fine – I didn't mean I needed the time off for me, it was to look after my wife.

No one offered me counselling. I'd have said no anyway. Move on, the world demanded, so I tried. I stopped talking to H about it, or anything related to it. I got worse by the week. I stopped eating, for the temporary illusion of having control over one aspect of my life.

Of course, it couldn't have helped that every single aspect of my work involved assisting women to fall pregnant, scanning their babies or delivering them. It helped even less that I was made to feel that my grief was neither genuine, nor worthy of attention. But this is the culture we live in, and ploughing-ahead-while-burying-all-the-things-you-can't-talk-about is a great healer. So that's what I did. Because that's what doctors always do.

Tick tock, tick tock, tick tock . . .

Chapter 17

I applied to run the London Marathon. Not to be its CEO, which might have been slightly less daunting, but to don a lycra leotard and actually haul myself round the fucker. My constant base-level guilt about leaving medicine occasionally erupts into having to do something vaguely useful for society. This usually means performing at a fundraiser, rather than doing a massive charity no-fun-run, but my subconscious must have been absolutely paralysed with guilt that day.

By way of context, I hadn't run since it was a mandatory school activity, enforced at starter-gunpoint. My approach to exercise in general was very much that of an autumn-years manatee. Even emergencies back on the ward would rarely involve more than a spirited waddle – a full-blown sprint would leave me unable to speak in full sentences by the time I arrived, let alone perform a caesarean. Me running a marathon is the equivalent of a normal person doing a round-the-world swim.

J insisted I speak to my spinal surgeon and my cardiologist, clearly keen to head off any kind of life-long-carer or coroner situation. This was probably a fair suggestion but one I ignored completely, and when questioned about it later, I lied that I'd been given a clean bill of health, both vertebral and ventricle. I'd signed up for a guaranteed charity place, through the St

John Ambulance. If I ended up being declared unfit to run, I imagined the guilt of pissing off a charity would far outweigh any discs or valves that might explode during the process.

In their confirmation email, they mentioned the 'unimaginable difference' my commitment would make to their vital work: every year they teach 800,000 people to save lives through their first aid training, and at the previous year's London Marathon alone, they treated 5,000 particitrousers for endurance-related maladies and mishaps. This year I was more than likely going to be one of them and while I'm sure they don't play favourites when scooping up slumped runners and wrapping them in tin foil, it clearly wouldn't do me any harm to have their logo on my vest.

Commitment made, I had just two items on my to-do list: 1) learn how to run a hundred miles, or however long it is, and 2) raise the £2,500 minimum charity donation. The idea of training didn't stress me out too much. I had somehow convinced myself that the marathon was merely a glorified walk in the park, which a propaganda coup had brainwashed the population into thinking was a huge feat. It made perfect sense – a multi-billion-dollar fundraising industry was predicated on this myth. A bit like how neurosurgery is actually no harder than a game of Operation but they want the big bucks so pretend it's super-complicated.★

Neither did the fundraising task worry me outrageously. After all, Barack Obama had raised $181 million from small donations and I only needed a thousandth of one per cent of that. I set up an online bucket-shaking page with Virgin

---

★ Hence the expression 'It's hardly brain surgery' – you can imagine them high-fiving one another at the Neurosurgery Marketing Board the day they came up with that.

Money, who immediately sent me an email which began: 'By now your training will be well underway.' Fear shot through me like Paula Radcliffe's intestinal contents onto a pavement. Time to start moving.

There was a running shop in Shepherd's Bush, approximately two miles away. I decided to limber up by quick-walking all the way there, stopping only once for a bottle of water and once to catch a bus because I was feeling a bit breathless. In store, I motored round the aisles like a wolf in a panini factory, bundling two of everything into my arms, until a lady came over to offer me a basket. She was wondering, based on my buying behaviour, if I'd happened to have signed up for the London Marathon. Presumably it was high season for this kind of thing, like a puppy shop the week before Christmas. She kindly rifled through my basket and removed everything I didn't actually need: a watch that monitored my heartbeat, a set of ladies' running tights (not sure what happened there) and a canister of dry shampoo. She also added some things I'd forgotten: a holster to strap my phone to my arm, a bum bag to humiliate me and a pack of plasters to slap over my nipples to avoid chafing them to a fine pâté. I was horrified to learn that this is apparently something that happens. I took a deep breath. All I could do now was focus on my training.

Focus is probably too strong a word for what transpired, but I did soon build up a daily routine that consisted of trotting round the block every morning when I got out of bed at the crack of lunchtime. As a result, initially unthinkable distances soon became, if not easy, then at least conceivable. The human body – even a discarded couch of a body such as mine – is an astonishing thing and I was routinely amazed that I'd made it home, still upright in my Asics rather than being wheeled in by a paramedic. As the weeks staggered by, I began to think, 'Maybe I can actually do this.'

I was feeling vaguely positive about the fundraising too, thanks in the main to Twitter. In an act of desperation and fear, I'd started posting my fundraising link to my followers with a promise that I would follow back every person who bunged me a pound or more. Bizarrely, the excitement of the implied virtual attention of a barely-known-former-doctor-turned-writer-and-comedian was a more glittering prize than I'd ever dared to imagine and, thanks to the genuine kindness of hundreds of online strangers, it resulted in a steady stream of charity income. Donations were mostly in the £5–10 bracket and they saw me comfortably over my target, for which I remain grateful to this day. Who said Twitter was all cancel culture and Nazis?*

I was particularly grateful to @███, a Twitter user, who'd pledged around half my remaining total in one go. A paltry followback didn't quite seem enough of a thank you for such a hugely generous gesture. It's a very weird feeling to receive an enormous chunk of cash from a total stranger, even if I was just a wheezy conduit for the donation, so it felt like the least I could do was to send over a big bouquet of flowers. J's appraisal of the situation – 'That's a terrible idea' – helped no one and was duly ignored.

Friends would ask what time I was aiming to finish in. Hang on, were they expecting me to . . . win? Wasn't it enough that I was taking part? If pushed, I'd plump for something round the five-hour mark, on the basis that gold medallists could knock one out in just over two hours.† The idea that they were

---

* It's only 99 per cent cancel culture and Nazis.

† 13mph! That's nearly the speed limit outside a school!

two-and-a-half-times faster than me seemed reasonable. But no more than that. Also, I realised you can walk the bloody thing in about six and a half hours, so anything over five was already picking at the seams of sponsorability.

Training went by in almost no time, mostly because I had almost no time to train. On marathon morning itself, I thought I'd be more nervous but J thoughtfully distracted me by initiating an enormous argument. He had decided it was unsafe for him to support me in person as he thought the marathon was a likely terrorist target. The term 'sitting duck' was used more than once. We eventually reached a mutually unhappy compromise where he would follow my progress on the website and turn up briefly at a pre-arranged point so I could stagger by and wave. My pulse had just about returned to normal by the time I took my place in the terrified crush of the marathon holding pen. I nervously fondled my bum bag which, for reference, contained:

- Enough jelly babies to keep a nurseryful of children hysterical for a fortnight. I had used my residual medical knowledge to calculate my calorie-per-mile requirements, in order to avoid being found by the side of a road like a soiled napkin. I then converted that calculation into rainbow-coloured gelatine newborns, like I imagine all proper athletes do.

- Spare nipple plasters. Obviously. No way was I leaving that shit to chance. The Mona Lisa has her smile, I have my nipples.

- Spare headphones. On my final training run, my headphones drowned in ear sweat and totally stopped working. I wasn't going to risk my own thoughts being my only accompaniment for an entire marathon.

There was a surprising amount of time spent hanging around awkwardly beforehand. Hundreds of us, scared little sausages shivering in fluorescent polyester. I got chatting to a friendly middle-aged man who was also running his first marathon. He explained he was doing it in memory of his friend who died during a marathon. This seemed odd to me, like playing Russian roulette in memory of a friend killed in a shooting. It also made me realise for the first time that reaching the other kind of finish line – the unhappy one in the sky – was even a possibility. Maybe I should have called the fucking cardiologist after all. But it was too late now – we were off.

First mile marker. Five jelly babies. A pleasing conduit for my calories: innately cheerful and slightly retro. Mile two. Five more jelly babies. I imagined an advertising campaign in which Bassetts establish the jelly baby as a symbol for the body positivity movement and this made me forget about the shooting pain in my lungs for almost an entire minute.

Mile markers were crucial – not just for jelly baby top-ups but also for keeping track of how much personal agonising torture was left, like checking the progress bar on a Liam Neeson film. By about mile ten, I was pretty much over jelly babies. By mile fifteen they were making me retch.*

J was lurking around mile seventeen, looking so nervous and shifty that I'm surprised he didn't end up in the back of an anti-terrorist unit van himself. I jogged on the spot as I spoke to him, worried that if I stopped moving my legs they might never start again, like a knackered boiler. I wheezed out how well it was all going; he flinched from the squeal of a nearby

---

* Years later, even writing about them is giving me acid reflux.

child and then we ran off in our separate directions at roughly the same speed.

What kept me going was the thought that if I didn't complete the race, I'd presumably have to pay back all the people who'd pledged money and organising the Refund of Shame sounded like a level of admin I could happily live without.

The bad news was I didn't win. Tsegaye Kebede pipped me to it in two hours and six minutes. The good news was I did complete the race both alive and under my notional five-hour target. I won't bother you with the details of quite how many minutes or hours faster. It's not a competition.

Crossing the finishing line came with the incredible sense of relief and achievement you'd imagine it would, although this was followed immediately by a feeling of pulverising anti-climax. Marathon staff expertly combined the exhilaration with the supreme pointlessness of it all in one swift movement, by giving me a gold medal plucked from an enormous card-board box containing literally tens of thousands of identical gold medals. Fool's gold.

I hobbled from the finish line to the St John Ambulance after-party where I drank flat prosecco like it was Zeus's own cum. A sign advertised a free sports massage – unfortunately, though, the massage table was upstairs and my legs let me know in no uncertain terms that stairs were off.

A couple of days lying in bed and a couple more generally complaining, and I was back to normal, which also involves a fair amount of lying in bed and complaining. Normal might not be the perfect word, actually – the next paragraph is an excerpt from a police witness statement because, annoyingly, J was right. Not about the terrorism.

Witness statement

. . . From that point onwards, I started to receive dozens of private Twitter messages from @ ▮ *in which she ultimately declared her love for me. I felt uncomfortable with this but was unsure of the best way to go about getting her to stop. This came to a head when Ms* ▮ *contacted me, asking me where I was on a night out. I didn't tell her where I was and sent a message making an excuse. Almost immediately, she started sending me further messages stating that I was evil and that I was trying to destroy her life. The following day, Ms* ▮ *sent a very long email to my personal email account. I refer to this email as exhibit AK/01 . . .*

Extract from Exhibit AK/01 – email correspondence

. . . Every part of me loves you and I know I can trust you more than anyone else. There is nothing I own that I would not just give to you in an instant, even if just to make you smile. I will never betray you or hurt you, no matter what happens. I sometimes forget how fast my mind works and the days are a blur, but I know that you are in my heart, it's like you always have been. . .★

It's fair to say I'm not normally the kind of person who generally receives declarations of love. That was the third. The first two were considerably easier to handle, having come from people I'd already consented to co-habit with. And, to be honest, neither of them were as fulsome as this one.

It felt ridiculous to even entertain the idea that I, a humble ex-doctor turned admittedly less humble writer-comedian, had acquired a stalker. I felt like the very opposite of a celebrity: I

★ I have slightly paraphrased these sections to keep the book under 500 pages.

didn't have a compound with huge iron gates or travel every-where in a Maybach. I lived in a two-bedroom flat and walked to the shops in my slippers. Even the gas board spelled my name wrong.* I didn't quite know what to do for the best, but I was fairly sure things weren't so bad that they couldn't be smoothed out by a well-worded email.

J told me to leave well alone, but that just seemed rude. There was also the possibility – unflattering as it was to my ego – that she was mentally unwell rather than truly infatuated by my charms. I just had to break the spell, gently. I needed to be kind and considerate, yet emphatic.

It's probably easiest if I disappear from your life as quickly as I appeared. Block me on Twitter if that makes it easier for you. Best, Adam.

Needless to say, this didn't do the trick. I should have known that it's pointless to apply rational thought to a situation fuelled by irrationality. I guess all she wanted was contact – not just attracting my attention, but holding it. The tone of my message was irrelevant, as were the contents: I could have written out the recipe to a Bombay Bad Boy Pot Noodle and still received in return the exact same 3,500-word reply. A reply that the police ended up calling 'Exhibit AK/02', but I call 'Holy Fuck'.

Extract from Exhibit AK/02 – email correspondence

. . . Thank you for being heartless, cruel and unkind just because you can. Thank you for throwing my trust, kindness and generosity right back at me, and for doing your utmost to totally destroy me. You will

------

* Thinking about it, if I was going to stalk someone, I reckon I'd probably aim nice and low too. Cardi B has a huge security detail, but what about the guy who does the dog voice on the Churchill adverts? Less of a scalp, sure, but a more achievable goal.

never hear from me again. If you had just been honest with me, you would never have heard from me in the first place . . .

I reasoned that while this clearly wasn't the calm resolution I had hoped for, it was at least some form of resolution. Taking to heart her promise to evaporate, like the lid of every pen I've ever owned, I blocked her on social media and instructed my email account to divert any future messages from her into the spam folder, alongside the weekly updates from a website where I bought a glue gun six years earlier. I paid my admirer no further thought, until I didn't have any option but to: she appeared to be in the early stages of recruiting an army.

Extract from Exhibit AK/03 – public Twitter interactions

From @▓▓▓ *to me:*
She may not be able to defend herself, which is clearly why you did it to her, but we can, whether she wants us to or not.

From @▓▓▓ *to @*▓▓*:*
I'm going to airport, DON'T make me have to come back here again. Tho I will of course, if needs be, we have address right? Text it to me.

Oh, come off it. No one had my address. Unless . . . doubts began to form. Had there been a return address on the flowers I'd sent? I asked my friend Tim, a lawyer. He reminded me that he was a lawyer, not a florist. Then he checked the registration data for my website and a free-to-use online electoral roll, and bingo – my exact whereabouts were splashed all over the internet. I might as well have hosted an open house.

And was this really some acquaintance of hers, who had my address and was champing at the bit to defend her honour?

Or was it my stalker herself, using a sock puppet account to intimidate me? I certainly wouldn't have bet against her in a fight; there are very few people in the country I'd be odds-on to beat – mainly very premature babies and the comatose.

Even if she didn't have my address, I was still extremely findable and killable. That night, for example, I was due to appear on stage at a well-publicised theatre event. The whole point of promotion is that your privacy is compromised when marketing requires it. Time for some logic – I'm not Justin Bieber but equally, this wasn't imaginary. Murders are rare, but it would be a dramatically satisfactory ending for the narrative arc of my life.

I talked it through with J, who went full scorched-earth and told me to pull out of all gigs until further notice. I politely explained that this was bananas. He then told me I had to hire a bodyguard. When I explained that this new solution was even more bananas, he insisted that I pull out of all gigs until further notice. We did a few laps of this conversation before I phoned the bodyguard agency.

The lady on the other end of the phone was extremely nice. They're actually known as close protection officers, she said. No, normally they'd wear everyday clothes, so as to be able to blend in, but yes, they'd be happy to wear a suit and sunglasses if I wanted. No, obviously they don't carry guns. Yes, they'd be able to drive me there and back. No, the car isn't bullet-proof. Yes, they have someone available. The cost for the evening would be £600 . . .

As much as I didn't want to be murdered, I was only getting £90 for the gig, so I explained to J that no close protection officers were available at such short notice. I assured him, however, that I'd be fine – I'd give the box office ██████'s name and let them know she was persona non grata insana. And if anyone came at me, I'd sprint off into the distance at my new top speed of 5.42 miles per hour.

It's difficult to tell who's out there when you're up on stage, what with all the theatre lights pointing at your face. You mostly just catch snapshot silhouettes of the audience – shoulders bobbing up and down, which hopefully means laughter, rather than choking to death on a Revel. Sometimes, however, conditions conspire through gaps in the lights and you get a lock on someone in the audience. At this show, the only person I could see between the lights was sat a few rows back, bang in the middle, a lady in her fifties with a disarmingly placid stare and the largest bouquet of flowers I have ever seen. As a consequence, my mind wasn't entirely on my material. This was her, right? Was she planning to storm the stage? Would it be soft kisses she rained down upon me or cold, hard blade-clutching fists? Was there a bread knife within the mixed chrysanthemums? I limped to the end of my set then ran off stage and straight to the tube, checking behind me like people do on the telly.

I asked Tim the lawyer if this situation had now become police territory. He said it definitely had, so the next morning I printed out a load of tweets and rehearsed in my head how to explain to a desk sergeant what Twitter was. As it happens, the officer I saw was actually very helpful and had even dealt with Twitter stalking in the past. While he didn't quite say, 'Well, I've never heard of you,' he did ask a lot of questions about which panel shows I'd been on, in the same way my mum does at Christmas. He took my statement and assured me that the lady in question would be contacted and kindly requested to stop with all the weird shit. Or words to that effect.

Witness Statement

Although the direct communication stopped, I was aware that Ms ▇▇▇▇ was continuing to talk about me on her Twitter feed. She was sending up to 300 tweets a day. The main theme of these tweets was that I'd made her ill and caused her to lose large amounts of money. She also tweeted that I had caused her dog to suffer from epilepsy.

Life went on, as it generally does. I would occasionally look at her Twitter account to see if she was still doing her thing. She always was – babbling away online about my fifty-faced awfulness and general lack of moral fibre. Or sometimes about how wonderful I was. Then a box arrived at my house.

Exhibit AK/06

A large cardboard box measuring approximately 1.5 metres and containing:

1. *Two boxes of chocolate, haphazardly gift-wrapped*

2. *A children's book, haphazardly gift-wrapped*

3. *A very large framed illustration of a rabbit, haphazardly gift-wrapped*

4. *A card with the message, 'Apologies, I had to wrap this in the dark!'*

5. *A second card with the message, 'To Adam, Happy Birthday beautiful!* For all the birthdays I missed and all those I will miss. Farewell, hello. Love, me xxxxx'*

6. *A poem entitled 'How Lucky I am'*

---

* I'm not beautiful by any metric, and my birthday was four months earlier.

7. A 19,000-word letter*

8. Two long, peculiar grey scarves.

I thought this probably tipped the situation into 'actually a bit much' territory, so I hid the box from J to stop him going fucknuts then, when he was at work, dropped it off at the police station.

'What do you think this scarf is?' asked the officer at the front desk, as he processed the batty booty. 'It looks like it's made of . . . animal hair?'

A second officer concurred. 'Cat hair,' he stated, like this was by no means the first cat-hair scarf he'd seen. You couldn't help but admire the craftsmanship – thousands of individual hairs all woven together. So painstaking, so precise. That said, it could only have been creepier if there were cat skulls hanging like bells at each end. The officers then discussed having a fresh, slightly sterner word with her, in the form of a harassment warning.

And with that, my brief experience of being the object of someone's unusual fascination faded away. It was always there in the background, though, like the underlying sting of a urinary tract infection halfway through a week of antibiotics.

I've thought a lot about how I could have acted differently, how it could have somehow stopped short of the cat-hair incident and how many of my attempts to 'do the right thing' only made matters worse. I found myself wondering whether J is actually over-anxious or if I'm under-anxious. 'Just promise me you'll never write about this and stir it all up again.'†

---

* By way of context, 19,000 words is about a quarter of the length of this book. Tim the lawyer had a skim through and told me I probably didn't want to read it, so I didn't. The letter, that is.

† It's him, right?

It didn't escape my notice that none of this would have happened if I was still working on labour ward. It hadn't occurred to me when I left medicine and chose 'writer' from my admittedly very short list of potential careers that I would end up putting myself into the public eye, with all that entails.

As a doctor, I'd be remembered by the odd patient but it felt very unlikely that, however upset they were with my clinical management, they would circumvent the usual complaints process and send parcels of matted animal hair to my house. My boundaries were fairly well-defined in the hospital cocoon but now they're open to interpretation. Am I the reader's friend? Does the transaction of the book purchase promise anything else? A chat over email? An invitation to my birthday party?★

My new life requires me to have a 'social media presence'. At best, I'm swapping slivers of myself for followers and likes. At worst, I'm opening myself up to dangerous levels of attention. Is it really worth it?

After a little soul-searching, I identified the real enemy and excised it from my life immediately. My trainers and lycra had a quick spin through the washing machine and were merrily packaged off to the nearest charity shop. I never ran again.

★   1) No. 2) No. 3) Probably not. 4) Absolutely not.

Chapter 18

As Britain's twelfth-best-known doctor,* I was now getting invited to give speeches at medical establishments. They varied from med schools to gaggles of junior doctors, all the way up to the 'royal colleges', the rather grandiose name given to the professional bodies that represent the different branches of the medical tree: paediatricians, pathologists, physicians, psychiatrists and pso on.

One evening, I found myself at the lectern in the dining hall of one such royal college, providing a slightly more harrowing after-dinner speech than they were perhaps hoping for. I reminded a couple of hundred consultants that just because they're senior and experienced, it doesn't mean they're any less vulnerable than the next human being. They have bad days like anyone else and they too need to make sure they have a solid support network behind them. Pricked, they bleed; isolated, they have just as much chance of going to pieces. I asked them

---

* The official ranking goes: the ones who appear on breakfast telly and talk about erectile dysfunction; the ones who do kids TV; the ones with less disgusting books; the ones who murder a bunch of innocents and land up on the front pages; then me. Then Dr Alban, who sang 'It's My Life'. Shit, I've just remembered Paul Sinha from *The Chase*. Thirteenth, then.

if their juniors would feel comfortable coming to them with a problem. When was the last time they took their team out for a bowl of pasta? That might be enough; the difference between a struggling junior doctor reaching out for help and a struggling junior doctor making a self-destructive life decision.

I told them the story of why I left medicine – the moment that still haunted my dreams and refused to let go. I left it to the end of my speech because it wipes me out every time: the emotional equivalent of running up Ben Nevis in flip-flops. My voice cracked as I relived the single most horrendous and harrowing moment of my life. You go into this job with the aim of seeing a healthy mum and a healthy baby in every case, and on this occasion I ended up with neither – and it was my fault. I explained how at my lowest ebb, no one gave me the support I needed – no one noticed how much I was struggling and no one cared when I told them. I reminded them that there will be numerous junior doctors working for them who also require that support, and they needed to be there for them. I gave them everything, ripped my heart out and stood before them bleeding, trembling and ashamed. I was met with the kind of absolute, mortified silence that Remembrance Sunday could only dream of – but they got it.

Their president gestured to me to stay on the stage. I presumed I was about to be presented with a bottle of whisky or some ceremonial trinket or other, so I prepared my most humble smile. Instead, the esteemed professor slid in next to me at the lectern, making me shuffle awkwardly to one side. He spoke the following words into the microphone: 'Thank you for this, Adam. I think it's important for me to add that this of course isn't everyone's experience. What I mean is . . . not everyone is cut out for the job.'

He patted me on the shoulder and I walked off stage to the

sound of awkward muttering, feeling pretty awful. Clearly I'd misunderstood what he'd said, right? He wouldn't have deliberately derided me after baring my soul like that, surely? But . . . there wasn't really any other way of interpreting it. Back at my table, I was seeking the solace of coffee and chocolate truffles when a couple of well-wishers approached and advised me not to listen to him. They agreed with me, they said.

I took three more chocolate truffles from the table to cheer myself up on the drive home, then stood up. The president smiled at me and walked over – he clearly didn't want to end the evening on a sour note so was going to apologise, or clarify what he meant. Maybe someone had had a word, maybe he'd worked it out for himself – either way, it was the right thing to do.

I prepared my most magnanimous face and said hello, calling him by his surname, obviously. He was the sort of doctor who likes to be so senior and unapproachable that you're not even allowed to know their first name – like Lord Voldemort. Or Morrissey. He clapped me on the shoulder and said, 'Maybe just stick to the funny stories in future?'

Was it that I'd cracked open medicine's most precious chestnut: don't rock the boat, even when you're safely on shore? Or was it that I'd pointed out to the emperor that his knob was out? Nobody likes to be told that the way things have always been done aren't the right way. Like the camera flash in *Get Out* that momentarily jolts the zombies out of their stupefaction,★ what if my talk had planted a seed of doubt in his audience? Or worse still, was it that I'd committed the cardinal doctorly sin and been honest about my feelings? With a curt nod that told

---

★ Sorry for another spoiler but it was released in 2017 and if you haven't seen it by now, you probably never will. You really should though, it's excellent.

– FLASHBACK –

Morrissey

It's always interesting to watch someone make the transition from senior registrar to consultant. Most of them manage to remain broadly the same person and maintain a degree of humility – they're aware that their new job title hasn't suddenly bestowed godlike therapeutic abilities upon them and stick to first-name terms with their junior colleagues. But some of them . . . don't.

Dr Octopus was a newly anointed consultant in a hospital I'd just started working at and was taking it all extremely seriously: monogrammed briefcase, stiff-looking suit and an absolute insistence on everyone using his surname. This was slightly weird for the nurses who'd known him as Chris for the past half-decade, but any time someone deadnamed him, he would urgently correct them. I've always felt that respect should be equal and mutual, rather than lopsided and built on weird neolithic conventions. Otherwise, it just increases the odds you'll do something you don't want to because you've been told to by some highfalutin surname-slinger. This can lead to poor clinical decisions and, in my case, when Dr Octopus asked me on a date, poor social ones.

Instead of feeling like I was being taken advantage of in

any way, I reasoned I was far too junior to say no to him.* So I said yes, hoping I'd work up the confidence to say no at a certain point in the evening without it becoming awkward. But would I? What if I ended up marrying the bloke?

Not to say it was the case with any of them, but I could think of a bunch of consultants married to doctors at least a decade younger. Love is love and age is no boundary, but at the same time, there was clearly a baked-in power imbalance from day one.†

Still, there were positives. Dinner with Dr O was bound to be nicer than the cheerless Lean Cuisine affair defrosting in my shared kitchen. Plus, it might mean I got shouted at slightly less on the wards. And last but not least, it's always interesting to find out what another person's penis looks like.

At first, dinner was a rather stilted affair. Any question I asked him seemed to get a single-word, often single-syllable reply, as if he was suddenly regretting letting this pleb peek under the hood of his life. I compensated by talking incessantly, like I was an auctioneer selling off random anecdotes. My conversational scattershot eventually hit its target, however, when I quizzed him about his consultant colleagues and realised he wanted to spend the entire evening slagging them off. Although there are few things quite as unattractive as watching someone parade

---

* I suppose using superiority to guarantee sexual congress is pretty much the first rule in the Harvey Weinstein playbook.

† The work of academia that best describes the medical hierarchy is *Blackadder* series three, episode three. Blackadder is annoyed, so he kicks the cat, which bites the mouse, which in turn bites Baldrick. And so the dominos tumble.

their insecurities by pushing other people down, at the same time it was brilliantly fascinating. I learned about the paediatric consultant who got through more ketamine than a stable of skittish thoroughbreds; the surgeon whose operating style was so slipshod that intensive care always made sure there was a bed spare if he was giving a patient so much as a haircut; the professor who demanded IT investigate why his computer was running so slowly, then had 'absolutely no idea' how all those nurses-in-bondage videos had found their way onto his hard drive.

By a certain point, the expensive alcohol had weaved its magic spell and I accepted the gossiping consultant's invitation to join him inside his house, then inside his bedroom, then inside his colon. Instead of a blissful afterglow, however, I had this sudden and overwhelming feeling that I'd made a horrible mistake. I should never have said yes to dinner, let alone this genital sharing. How on earth did I think this was going to improve work relations? I decided, under the circumstances, the best thing I could do was to get out and get home, so I made my excuses.

'I'm really sorry, Chris – I've got an early start in the morning. I should probably get home.' His brow furrowed. He was annoyed. Did he want me to stay? Did he want to sweetly spoon me all night and make me huevos rancheros in the morning?

'Sorry,' he said. 'Do you mind if we stick with "Dr Octopus"?'

Chapter 19

When a letter arrived from the Secretary of State in a fancy ivory-coloured envelope with a portcullis on the front, there was a moment where I genuinely impressed myself.★ If I was suddenly run over by a skip lorry, it might be noteworthy enough to make it into a local paper.

It was from Jeremy Hunt, the then-Secretary of State for Health who, aware of my book *This is Going to Hurt*, wondered if I'd like to pop in for a chat. That he was aware of my book didn't surprise me, considering the number of people at book readings who'd asked me to sign a couple of copies – one I'd make out to Aunt Julia, wishing her a quick recovery after her hip replacement, and a second one to Jeremy Hunt. Plus there was the fact that the book ended with an open letter to Mr Hunt, where I accused him of being supremely out of touch, callous, and disrespectful to NHS staff.

It wasn't immediately clear what he hoped to achieve from

★ The only previous such time was when I was half a mile back in a queue for a gig and an excited, clipboard-wielding PR person rushed up to inform me that there was a VIP entrance. My ego boost deflated faster than a sex doll on a stag do when the PR had realised her mistake. Slightly ashen-faced, she re-inserted me four people from the back of the queue, explaining that she'd mistaken me for the singer from early noughties minor pop-rock sensation Good Charlotte.

our meeting but two options presented themselves as the most likely. Either he wanted to change my mind and somehow persuade me that he was, in fact, against all the evidence I'd presented, a kind, empathetic, reasonable man with the best interests of junior doctors shot through him like a stick of rock. Or he wanted to tear me limb from limb and feed my freshly pulled flesh to the lake of emperor scorpions I imagine he keeps as pets. Alternatively, perhaps he just wanted me to take six hundred signed copies of my book off his hands.

I agreed to the meeting immediately, then spent the intervening week working out what to say to him, plus gently getting my affairs in order. Richmond House in Westminster was a lot less fancy than I thought it would be – in my head, the address conjured the august majesty of Whitehall crossed with the riverside splendour and bizarre snootiness of Richmond-upon-Thames. In the architect's head, however, it conjured a Travelodge off junction 9 of the M40.

I was ushered into the ministerial office, where I shook Mr Hunt's hand, accepted a glass of water that didn't overtly smell of strychnine and sat down on the sofa. Then I pulled out the piece of paper I'd written my questions and scraps of data on, and got stuck in.

I started by asking if he was happy that he'd accused hard-working doctors of striking for money, when in reality they were simply protesting an unfair new contract which was being imposed on them and they knew would jeopardise patient safety.

It's slightly demoralising to meet someone with whom you disagree absolutely and profoundly on an ideological level, who then has the gall to be cleverer than you. It was like playing tennis against a pro – this question, and everything else I lobbed at him, however perfectly aimed and well-practised, was volleyed back and thudded right onto my baseline with no hope of me reaching it. Not only had he gone to a far more expensive school than me, he'd clearly opted for the debating society instead of saxophone lessons. Plus, I realised, he must have faced every single one of these questions many, many times before. But I kept asking, trying to pull a point back in the match.

Eventually, he got pissed off with me and my questions – 'I thought I'd invited you in for a nice chat, not an interview' – which was fair. I did try to explain that no one ever said that the chat had to be nice, but the damage was done and the atmosphere was very much like I'd set fire to some ministerial paperwork before daubing a Hitler moustache made from my own faeces onto the portrait of the Queen.

At one point, I thought I saw him slyly press a button under the table, as if I was going to be trapdoored into the scorpion lake, but that was probably my imagination. A few seconds later, one of his juniors just happened to pop by to remind Mr Hunt that his next meeting was about to start. He might as well have teamed it with a theatrical wink. Either way, I took the hint and stood up to take my leave. Nemesis or not, I somehow felt the need to apologise. I tapped the copy of my book which I'd brought along. 'I'm sorry if I came across nicer on paper than I do in real life.' The minister considered this as he shook my hand. 'Oh no,' he replied. 'I think you've been quite consistent.'

I spent the tube journey home coming up with brilliant retorts I wished I'd said at the time, mostly along the lines of, 'Go fuck yourself, you serpent. Do you even care how much blood there is on your hands from the cuts you introduced?'★

★ You are welcome to read Mr Hunt's account of his time in office. *Zero* is available for £20 RRP, and has sold 1,800 copies at time of press.

If we measure a Secretary of State for Health by the number of needless deaths they cause – sadly, the standard unit of measurement in their profession – Jeremy Hunt's successor, Matt Hancock, was even worse. Not for waging a war against junior doctors but rather for waging a war against science and common sense, apparently hoping that a virus that behaved utterly predictably in every country in the world would some-how be stopped in its tracks in the UK, by good old British spunk and a dash of Blitz spirit.

I went to Hancock's office★ a couple of times and he actually seemed a nice enough bloke. Speaking to him, I never felt that I was being bested in a game of intellectual tennis but nor did I have the suspicion he wanted to nail my testes to the central plinth of Westminster Bridge. The first time I visited, he was freshly inserted into his new position, having formerly been the Paymaster General, then in charge of the Department of Digital, Culture, Media and Sport – a system no weirder than if the new England football manager used to be the Archbishop of Canterbury and then before that, Lulu.

The previous night, I'd been performing in the West End and was struck by the presence of a large poster in my dress-ing room informing me that if I, or anyone working in the theatre, had any stresses whatsoever – emotional, financial, work-related, home-related – then we could call a free, 24/7, union-funded helpline, which would provide immediate sup-port and counselling as and when required. I told him that no such equivalent poster supporting doctors existed in any UK hospital. If you're struggling, then generally the best you can attempt is to contact occupational health, who, in the absence

★   Or sex palace, as it later turned out to be.

of any set rulebook about what to do next and in the probable absence of a counsellor to whom to delegate, might suggest a bit of time off. What's even more likely, however, is that they'll chat to the consultant you were too afraid to speak to yourself and between them they'll recommend you bite the bullet and muddle through, stiff upper lip and all that. Matt Hancock told me that this didn't sound right at all and promised that someone from his office would be in touch to outline the systems of which I was merely unaware but which he had no doubt were definitely in place. An email came back a few days later, basically saying, 'Shit! You're right!'

Rather amazingly, a couple of months after this, Matt Hancock launched a helpdesk for doctors, hugely expanding on what had been a London-only service for GPs and making it available to all species of doctors, across the country. He even name-checked my book in his announcement, which was unnecessarily good of him. As this would make a genuine difference to my former colleagues, I decided to slightly lay off the guy when he was next doing his rounds of specious politicianing. I mean, he'd almost certainly saved the lives of doctors with this intervention, and that was to be commended.

And then Covid happened. As the virus swept through Europe and lapped at our shores, I became very vocal online and off, sharing my views that Matt Hancock and the government were fucking up across the board and that as a result of their inaction, people were going to die. The horrendous news reports coming from Italy of body bags streaming out of hospitals were going to be us in a fortnight unless we did something dramatic; our nursing homes were becoming Covid breeding grounds before our very eyes; we were negating our island advantage by inviting practically anyone in, the more virulent the better; and the backdoor plan was clearly for everyone to catch the disease and confer herd immunity on a herd that would end up culled to the tune of millions. I didn't claim to be any kind of virology Nostradamus – I was just looking at the data and listening to my friends, family and colleagues working in hospitals and GP practices. Not much perhaps, but still something that the government was singularly failing to do.

I didn't change anyone's mind, sadly. But I did piss off Matt Hancock, who began sending me direct messages on Twitter. It started with flattery.

'If you'd like a briefing on our approach then please ask. As a significant influencer, I am keen to ensure you have the scientific facts.'

Then he turned it up a gear, trying to worry me that I would cause actual harm.

'I've already had journos in touch re your tweet saying "Adam says you're not doing enough". But doing (a) the wrong thing or (b) the right thing too soon makes things worse . . . Please please don't just call for action and give the populists cover!'

I replied to suggest that he was heading towards option (c) – doing the right thing too late. This sadly and needlessly proved to be the case, as tens of thousands of bereaved family members can attest.

As we stood on our doorsteps and clanged our pans, politicians were handing out billion-pound contracts to their mates. As we put rainbows in our windows, nursing home residents were being all but murdered by their idiotic policies. And throughout, as NHS staff put their lives at risk, as they worked double and triple shifts, as the PPE cut into their faces, as they moved out of their family homes for months on end, the ghouls in charge seemed far more concerned with their own appearances and legacies. And there's still nothing approaching an assurance that the NHS won't be sold off in five years' time, plunging us into an unfair insurance-based system that mostly benefits the former politicians who stuff the boardrooms of private medicine.

Matt Hancock continued to reply privately whenever I said anything negative about him or his pronouncements, one day dropping all pretence when I called him out on some weasel words and just saying 'Grateful if you could remove that tweet.' Two-hundred-and-fifty-four people died of Covid that day and he seemed more interested in cleansing his social media timeline.

Maybe he thought we had a mutual understanding, I don't know. Equally, I knew I could use this powerful connection to do good things – did I really want to sever it? But he was asking me to censor myself to give him an easier ride – it felt grimy. And if I did, then what might he ask me to do next – feed me spin to put out into the ether?

I asked J, who told me I had to send that to a newspaper. Surely trying to silence people who disagree with you doesn't fit into the ministerial job description, he argued.* I convinced myself that it was too minor for anyone to be interested in printing, plus it might be illegal to show a message from someone without their permission. Besides, I had so much work on I didn't really want to distract myself. But the truth was I'd been conditioned not to make a fuss.

---

* And then, when he heard on the radio that land might have to be compulsorily purchased for use as graveyards, became convinced that this would happen to our garden and spent the rest of the day pacing about and trying to work out which patch of lawn he would miss the least.

Hancock* was no different to the consultants and clinical directors I'd met in the NHS – dressing up the suppression of individual thought as 'for the common good'. It was beaten into me that the way to succeed in the NHS was to be quiet and mediocre, to never stick your hand up, and that takes a lot of unlearning. The minister slid out of my direct messages just as effortlessly as he slithered into them. The tweet stayed exactly where it was, but I kept it all quiet. Well, until I published it in this book.

---

* His successor, Sajid Javid, wrote to me to say his wife enjoyed *This is Going to Hurt*. Cute, but maybe you should read it, mate?

His successor, Steve Barclay, was appointed the week before this book was printed, but I'm not convinced he can read, and will probably be out of a job by the time this hits the shelves.

Chapter 20

Prior to attending university, I don't believe I'd spoken to a single undergraduate student. This meant that everything I knew about students I'd learned from the TV show *University Challenge*, so I was convinced that university life consisted of bad hair, migrainous knitwear and highly charged whispering.*

University Challenge was one of the few shows we watched as a family and, I think it's fair to say, we took it seriously. I even went as far as printing out scorecards so we could compete against one another. How normal! A winning score usually involved getting four or five correct answers in half an hour of quickfire questioning and, much to my lower-wattage (although, in fairness, much younger) siblings' annoyance, I found myself on the victorious sofa most weeks. A few short years later, in my first year of university, I saw a poster recruiting for the medical school's *University Challenge* team and, exhibiting a really quite impressive level of cognitive dissonance, convinced myself that I might be up to the task. The written try-out proved quite conclusively that I shouldn't be allowed anywhere

---

* In fact, it also consists of beer, a fresher having a meltdown in the first week and her dad having to drive eight hours to come and get her, and the Christian Society making a demented quantity of toast.

near the show and I'd be better off with something less taxing, such as a word search in the *Beano*.

However, if there's one thing I've learned from getting ankle-deep in the peripheries of celebrity, it's that having an IQ lower than the freezing point of water in Fahrenheit★ is no barrier to getting what you want. All I had to do to achieve my starter for ten was play the long game, write a disgusting memoir and suddenly – twenty years down the line – the producers would come crawling back on bended forelocks offering me a place on their Christmas special. Rather than actual students, each university would be represented by four 'notable alumni'. The term 'notable alumni' was used so they didn't perjure themselves by writing the word 'celebrity',† which clearly neither applied to myself nor 90 per cent of the previous particitrousers who they dangled as bait.

There would be three rounds: a first round filmed in late November, with the semi-finals and final taking place on a second date in December. I would have to commit to both dates, which I was happy to do. The truth was, I'd be on holiday for the second date (and I don't think either the travel insurance or J would count this as reasonable grounds for cancellation) but I had enough insight into my lack of ability to be pretty confident I wouldn't make it to the finals.

To give myself more of an idea about what to expect, I watched one of the 'notable alumni' specials from a previous series and was shocked to discover how much more cleverer I'd become over the years, answering over ten questions correctly! Impressive compared to my childhood scores, yes, but

---

★ 32 degrees. See, that's an easy five points.

† 'Celebrity is a mask that eats into the face' is a quote by which American novelist? That's right! John Updike. Another five points.

thankfully not impressive enough to jeopardise my holiday.*

'Guess which TV programme I'm appearing on?' I asked my dad.

'What have you done now?' he replied, no doubt presuming my rather unexpected public ascent had attracted the attention of a Channel 5 show called *Britain's Most Dangerous Doctors* or something else that might bring the family into further disrepute. On hearing the middle-class safe word of *University Challenge*, he became the most excited I've seen him outside of the occasional time when West Ham has won a match or a grandchild has arrived.

He went straight into full-on Tiger Dad training mode, telling me I needed to bone up on my motorways, the dates of all the key wars† and the greatest hits of the major British poets. Please could I make sure to get the medical questions right – and if I didn't, to at least drop round a vial of cyanide on my way back from taping the show because he wasn't sure he could cope with that level of embarrassment.

He asked how long I had to revise – a couple of months – and then told me it should be OK if I started now. He asked me who wrote *Dombey and Son* and then sighed deeply at my answer.‡ It was nicely nostalgic of preparing for my medical school interview. Two days later, a package arrived with a book of quotations and a set of flashcards about countries of the world.

---

* I then watched an episode of the real *University Challenge* and found myself once again drowning in a sea of ignorance. When it comes to their 'notable alumni', they clearly make the questions a lot easier.

† The Second World War lasted from 1st September 1939 until 2nd September 1945, an irrationally irritating six years and one day. Five points.

‡ Dickens – not, it turns out, Beatrix Potter. Although I maintain she'd have made a bloody good go of it. Nil points.

I didn't revise anything. Well, aside from anything else, I wasn't free for the final.

In the sitcom version of my life, I would go on the show, ace every question and drive my fellow notables into a commanding lead, then, rather than cancel my holiday, end up throwing the match by interrupting question after question with deliberately wrong answers. In the actual version of my life, I received an email from the producers not long before filming began, informing me that they had been unable to find four notable people who used to go to my university, meaning my invitation had to be rescinded.*

I called my dad to let him know the good news that he was spared the embarrassment of me being unable to identify the Moonlight Sonata or the Isthmus of Tehuantepec.† He sound-ed disappointed – he said he'd told lots of his friends that I was going to be on it.

'Even though you knew I'd be terrible?'

'Because I'm proud of you.'

In a two-minute interchange where we expressed more emotions to each other than in the previous four decades com-bined, I told him that meant a lot. He told me he was sorry medicine wasn't the right job for me – he only wanted me to do it because he hoped I would love it as much as he did. I apologised that it didn't work out, and then he pretended it was time for his dinner and we never spoke of it again.‡

---

* I eventually discovered the full story: one of my teammates would have been weatherman turned climate change denier, future Covid naysayer and brother of Jeremy, Piers Corbyn. No one was prepared to share a desk with him.

† Yes, it's in Mexico. ¡Cinco puntos!

‡ He certainly couldn't have given less of a shit when I appeared on an episode of Celebrity Pointless. Sadly, the channel cut the following exchange:
Richard Osman: Do you watch many films, Adam?
Me: Mostly Bisney and porn.

– FLASHBACK –

Starter For Ten

'I have always wanted to do medicine because it combines my long-held interest in the sciences with an ability to help people, and . . . '

Over and over and over, I parroted the magic words that would get me into medical school. My answers had been carefully prepared – not by me, but rather by a floating committee of stakeholders in my success: my parents, my parents' friends and colleagues, and my teachers. And this was my day of reckoning. Doors were set to automatic and I was cleared for take-off: it was interview time.

I shuffled into the waiting room repeating my mantra. 'I have always wanted to do medicine because it combines my long-held . . . '

'Kay!'

I meerkatted to attention and quickly scanned the room to see who'd just barked my name at Boeing decibels. Fucksake. Draped across a Chesterfield was Logan Howlett, as pleasant a sight as a toilet bowl full of blood.

'Howlett . . . How's it going?'

'You know each other?' asked one of the other three students, trembling like he had a pneumatic drill hidden somewhere deep inside him. No, we just randomly guessed each other's names.

Howlett looked so utterly at home, he may as well have been wearing slippers and a smoking jacket. 'Yeah, Kay's at Dulwich with me. Whizz at the old piano. What's your blazer?'

God grant me the confidence to talk to strangers like that. What a joy it must be to walk through any door and be able to hold your own no matter who you find on the other side. On second thoughts, god grant me the ability to mute the Howletts of this world so I can sit in silence and learn my answers. 'I have always wanted to do medicine because it combines my long-held interest in the sciences . . . ' Memorising my incantation wasn't particularly difficult; it was the sincerity I was struggling with. It was a lie, but a necessary one. The truth – 'I have never wanted to do medicine, but I have always been expected to' – might not go down quite so well.

It's only natural, I guess, for humans to have a vested interest in the future of their kids. From what I can see, most parents hope their children find something they love, something they really want to do and are good at; preferably something that isn't injecting heroin into their genitals in the backroom of a flat-roofed pub. Ideally, they'd then end up doing that beloved thing for a living, earn enough money to buy a nice house and visit every Sunday with their own charming offspring. My parents weren't most parents.

I was at school when I first realised that I much preferred playing the musical instruments I was learning to tick the boxes for my medical school application than the idea of medicine itself. When I suggested to my mum that perhaps I could go to music college, she reacted like I'd just announced I was marrying the cat.

'And become what?' she cried. 'A saxophone teacher?'

Well, yes actually – that sounded great. But apparently it was out of the question.

Soon Howlett was chairing a panel of the five of us, in a tightly monitored discussion about our backgrounds. Our schools, mainly. Of the five of us there, four were from private schools. Only one of us, Peggy, was from a state school.★

'Bit weird more people here went to the same private school than *any* state school?' said Peggy. But I'm not sure it was actually weird, though: it's a system deliberately designed to perpetuate medicine as the province of the posh. Half an hour later, I'd be telling the interview panel about the work experience I undertook in a hospital – work experience that was mandatory for all applicants. What would remain unsaid, however, was how much easier it is to blag a fortnight shadowing a surgeon when your parents' best friends are surgeons: forever dining together, playing bridge and smearing fox guts on each other's faces.

After I'd told them about the work experience, the panel would ask about my extra-curricular interests and I'd detail my accomplishments on the saxophone, piano, trombone and ever-handy harpsichord – something, it's safe to say, not every school has at their disposal. If the interview panel wanted even more proof of my apparent suitability, I could then bang on about my school concerts at the Royal Albert

---

★ Or 'the maintained sector', as it was sniffily referred to at our non-maintained school.

Hall or my knowledge of viniculture.* Everything about my schooling was privileged. I'd wanked in Shackleton's boat, for god's sake.†

Logan Howlett didn't particularly care for the idea that his presence in the room was less to do with his competence and more to do with the crest on his cufflinks, so he made a spirited but unconvincing defence to Peggy that he was absolutely there on merit and merit alone. She flashed him a smile that you didn't need a £4,000-a-term education to translate as 'get to fuck'. I didn't particularly care for the idea that I wasn't there on my own merits either – no one does – but at least I had the sense to keep my mouth shut.

Despite myself, I felt slightly defensive. I couldn't deny that doors had been opened for me but I'd definitely put in the work once I'd walked through them. The ceaseless studying, the endless after-school classes, the timetable of extra-curricular activities that would give any Olympic athlete a nervo. Not everyone at my school worked hard – I knew loads of pupils who were phoning it in, killing time until they got to the serious business of failing every exam and walking straight into a job in their daddy's shipping firm. So no, compared to those fuckers, I was there on merit.

Privilege is terrible, of course. It's deeply unfair. But I

---

* Every Friday evening from the age of sixteen, we had wine tasting lessons. This feels like it should result in the police seizing the teacher in question's hard drives, but at the time it was obviously amazing.

† Perched on some rocks in the north cloister of my school was this big old wooden boat, donated by some long-dead explorer who used to study there. At lunch and break times, whoever got to the boat first would pull back the cloth cover from the hatch and sit inside for some undisturbed time with their Blue Riband and Kia-Ora. Or worse.

was a good guy. Privileged, but good – it happens. Also, I was going to use my advantage to help people, like Mother Teresa or Spider-Man. Right. I rolled my shoulders, stuck out my chin and, as I was called to the interview, I smiled at Peggy to let her know that I was one of the good ones. She quarter-smiled back, like I was a child who'd just shown her the contents of his potty. Then I walked into the interview room with my head held high. I'd earned this.

'Kay!' bellowed an angular middle-aged doctor in a tweed jacket. 'Good to see you. You're Stewart's son, right?'

Chapter 21

While Paxman was tutting away in the *University Challenge* final, I was sat on a Miami toilet. As my blood pooled on the floor, my mind went slightly unhelpfully back to a question in my medical school interview. 'Why do so many people die on the toilet?' At the time, I felt like reminding them that I hadn't actually been to medical school yet, so how about they let me in and I'd get back to them in six years? Presumably there's some benefit to asking questions like this – perhaps it mines a certain aspect of logic and lateral thinking that only the finest future doctors will be able to access. Back then, it just felt like a meaningless way to humiliate me, like if they'd asked me to draw a horse using a Cumberland sausage.

I hesitantly offered up that the toilet might be where someone is more likely to head when they're feeling unwell, having underestimated exactly how unwell they are. They all looked at me with a mixture of disdain and pity.

My only other thought that seemed in any way relevant was that scene in *Jurassic Park* where a man is innocently curling one out when he's eaten whole by a rampaging T-Rex. I managed to keep that one to myself. Oh, wait – Elvis! Drugs! Yes! Junkies lock themselves in toilets and overdose? Surely. Another sad shake of the head, this time accompanied by a narrowing of the eyes. Was I a drug addict as well as a numbskull?

The tweed-clad member of my firing squad took pity on me. 'What happens when people strain?'

'Of course!' I replied. 'If they strain too hard, they might burst . . . ' I ran out of words – the noun I was looking for evaporated.

Taking pity once more, or perhaps worried that I was about to say ' . . . their anus', the nice man stepped back in. 'An aneurysm, yes. Well done.'

And then, the best part of two decades and several thousand uneventful intestinal evacuations later, I was having my own toilet-based emergency.

We had just checked out of our hotel room but still had twelve hours to kill before the flight home, so filled this dead air by hanging out by the pool. As I settled myself on the toilet seat for a restorative pre-swim poo, I felt something land on my head. Not wanting the last hours of my holiday to be marred by some kind of frightful Floridian insect laying eggs in my hair, I instinctively batted it away with my hand. Immediately, blood began to gush down my face onto the floor and my medical training informed me that it probably hadn't been an insect after all. I spotted that on the wall behind the toilet there was a broken picture frame, out of which a biscuit-sized triangle of glass had fallen. In brushing it away, the glass had sliced deep through the ring finger knuckle of my right hand.

The amount of blood, totally out of proportion with the size of the injury, suggested I'd sliced into some kind of small artery, the name of which I'd presumably known at some point. When I squeezed my knuckle with my other hand, blood just spurted through my fingers like an out-of-control fire hose in a cartoon. It went everywhere – onto my t-shirt, into my eyes, onto my bare legs and groin,★ all over the cubicle. I wrapped my finger in toilet roll but it was like trying to mop up the Mediterranean with a raffle ticket. Anxious not to become yet another death-on-a-toilet statistic, I managed to pull up my blood-stained trunks and stagger from the cubicle, my hand now wrapped in an eight-inch boxing glove of paper towels.

From the screams of the sunbathing families I passed on my way over to J, you'd have thought they'd never seen a man totally drenched in his own blood before. I might have expected a little less uproar from the land of near-daily mass shootings.

J took one look at me staggering towards him like Carrie on prom night and informed me, calmly, that we would be going to a hospital and I was not going to argue. Even though I was pretty sure I could sort it out with a few more minutes of firm pressure, I could also see J's point of view. Nice as it was that my blood was getting to enjoy the mock-marble pool copings, it would be better off remaining inside my body. A member of staff wandered over to confirm that he was also very much on board with the idea of me fucking the fuck away from his hotel, which was looking increasingly like a scene from *Nightmare on Elm Street 6: Pool Party*.

J bundled me into a cab, on the grounds that it'd be quicker than waiting for an ambulance, and we sped off to hospital with my hand wrapped in enough towels that the blood would never be able to seep through onto the upholstery. Or if it did, I'd definitely have bled to death by then, so I wouldn't be too concerned about a cabbie getting crabby.

★ Had my balls had a little 'holiday trim'? Let me just say this: the clippers were on my scrotum like a wolf on its favourite kind of toasted sandwich.

After taking my name and date of birth, the hospital's next question was how I was going to pay for my care. Which was reasonable, I guess. They were running a business after all, albeit a somewhat morally repugnant one. J happily informed them that of course we had holiday insurance: we were responsible adults, for heaven's sake. Then he handed back to me for the details. Instead of the policy number everyone was hoping I'd magic out of my swimming trunks, all I could offer up was that my insurance was provided as a free service through my bank. The receptionist looked at me like I'd just offered to pay them in teabags and suggested they take a swipe of my credit card 'just in case'. I could always get reimbursed by my 'insurer' at a later date. J immediately tried to have a fight with me about the very real possibility that we might be in the midst of a turbulent foreign issue that brought with no insurance, but I was still bleeding quite dramatically so I postponed the argument by responding in the weediest voice I could muster.

When you're an NHS patient, all you usually have to worry about is the issue that brought you in, plus perhaps whether there's a vegan option on the hospital menu. There's an extra frisson to being a patient in America: whether you'll survive, and whether you'll still have a house to go back to. The doctor asked if I wanted an X-ray of my hand. This would be standard practice back home to ensure that no glass had found its way into the joint – but it would set me back another thousand dollars, so they have to ask . . . Also, did I want the wound closed with surgical glue or stitches? Glue would give a better cosmetic result, but it was much more expensive. I felt like I was being upsold Scotchgard on a sofa. (I went for the cheapskate options and resigned myself to never being able to work as a hand model.)

I didn't envy the doctors either. Having to bring cost into

the equation when advising patients just doesn't feel . . . proper, and I'm enormously thankful I never had to do it during my medical career. Whatever the NHS's failings, there's no fairer way to decide who to treat than 'everyone' and no better way to treat them all than 'equally'. Meanwhile, in the US, health-care is not a human right but a commodity to be haggled over with insurance companies.*

Soon I was patched up, alive and sitting by a departure gate at Miami International, waiting for group fifteen to be called. My phone rang – it was the hospital with the line nobody wants to hear, 'I'm afraid it's not good news.' Happily, it was only financial bad news. Unhappily, this meant the cost of our holiday had more than doubled. My bank had denied any and all knowledge of the existence of my travel insurance policy. Weirdly, the student bank account that I opened in 1998 no longer carried its free holiday insurance perk the thick end of two decades later.

J was giving me the full hairdryer treatment as we walked off the land of the not-so-free and onto the plane and was still going as we whizzed over Iceland. He was curious to know how I could have passed my medical exams and yet still be 'so incredibly fucking stupid'. 'Think what we could have bought with that money! A year's shopping!'

I eventually shut my eyes and claimed I was feeling exhaust-ed due to blood loss. 'Look,' I said, 'it was your idea to take me to hospital.'

---

* The availability and affordability of healthcare remains Americans' num-ber one concern in poll after poll, with two thirds of US bankruptcies having healthcare bills as a contributory factor. Less than half of Americans can afford an unexpected medical bill of a thousand dollars, which, if my experience in Florida is anything to go by, probably wouldn't cover much more than a couple of Nurofen and a Band-Aid.

Chapter 22

My parents were coming to stay. It was the first time they'd been at ours for Christmas and the first time they'd ever stayed overnight somewhere we'd lived. Not through any kind of snub, it was just the first time we'd had a spare room and a dining table capable of hosting more than two people and a bottle of Mateus Rosé.

J likes to be liked, but he likes to be loved even more, so he treated it as a royal visit and spent a fortnight turning the previously empty spare room into far and away the most luxurious part of the house: ordering enough furniture, bedding and electric heaters to single-handedly send Jeff Amazon to Jupiter, and generating enough cardboard waste to keep the recycling bins full until we're both long dead. Every moment he wasn't wielding an Allen key was spent in the kitchen, working on a bafflingly complicated series of menus that would make Raymond Blanc give up and order a Deliveroo.

'You don't need to impress them,' I told him.

'I'm not trying to!' he said, before asking if he should do a twenty-five or a thirty-layer croquembouche.

The night before they arrived, I was performing in Brighton. After my soundcheck, I got a panicked text from J, instructing me to urgently source a duvet — it was apparently missing from

ADAM KAY

his order. I didn't reply, so this was followed up with a relatively antsy phone call, reminding me that this would represent my only contribution towards getting ready for Christmas.* I promised him that I'd do my best, so asked the helpful lady on the stage door where I might be able to find such a thing at 7 p.m. on a Thursday evening. She suggested a nearby TK Maxx.

I checked Google Maps to make sure I could get there and back before I was needed on stage. I could, just. When I arrived at TK Maxx less than ten minutes later, they did indeed have duvets among the designer jumble – more expensive than I'd have liked, but I was very much in the role of beggar rather than chooser. As I pegged it to the theatre, I took a few seconds to feel pleased with myself and imagine J's face as he smoothed out its luxurious togs and told me I'd 'saved Christmas'. With moments to spare, I wheezed back into the venue smugly sporting a king-size duvet. The lady on the stage door beamed at me indulgently.

'Oh, what a sweetheart you are!' she declared. My smile froze onto my face. I am, yes, but . . . I am? 'You bought that for the homeless man who sleeps outside the box office, didn't you? Would you like me to give it to him?'

I had the shortest moment to parse the options in my head. Do I put her straight and say I have absolutely no intention of helping the homeless man shivering pitifully in the doorway outside, just a couple of days before Christmas? Or do I cement my seconds-old reputation as a decent human being, and go along with the misunderstanding? As the Tannoy crackled to life and announced that patrons should take their seats immediately, my frozen smile thawed and I handed over the duvet without another word.

---

* Which was actually very unfair, as I'd also bought the Chocolate Oranges.

I sat down at the book-signing trestle table after the show and picked up a Sharpie.

'Hi, thanks for coming! Who can I make it out to?' [Remark about doctors' handwriting] 'Yeah, haha, it's the last thing that goes . . . '

'Hi, thanks for coming! Who can I make it out to?' [Remark about doctors' handwriting] 'Yeah, haha, it's the last thing that goes . . . '

'Hi, thanks for coming! Who can I make it out to?'

'You've forgotten me already?'

I looked up to see a teddy bear of a man. The rumpled shirt, scruffy hair and bottle of wine made me assume it was the homeless guy who'd stolen my duvet. He smiled broadly and I realised exactly who he was – Mike Schachter, the guardian angel who'd struck up a conversation with a shy eighteen-year-old and changed his life. He said he'd been watching my career with interest and had told numerous medical students to read my books. 'I've come for my commission,' he added.

I asked what had changed at the medical school in the last twenty years. Staff had come and gone, buildings had been constructed and demolished, but the stuff that students were taught, and more importantly not taught, unfortunately sounded about the same – his pastoral services were still very much required. Our reminiscences were interrupted by a punter stood by the ice creams loudly pointing out quite how long the queue was, so I apologised and made a mental note to misspell his name when he reached the front. I hugged Mike awkwardly over the trestle table and I told him he shouldn't have bought a ticket. 'Ahh, you weren't that bad!' he said, and lolloped off.

I was still smiling when I drove home. Crawling into bed, I casually explained my lack of duvet to J with a dopey grin, hoping he might join in with the sitcom theatrics and shake his head lovingly, while simultaneously pinching my cheek and saying, 'Oh, *you.*'

Instead, he called me a fucking idiot and asked me why I didn't stop off at the twenty-four-hour Tesco in Earl's Court on my way back home. Driving there at 4 a.m.* on Christmas Eve, I asked myself the same question.

---

* One advantage of nightmaring awake in the middle of the night is that you can avoid the traffic.

Chapter 23

There really needs to be some kind of gay starter pack for new arrivals. It would obviously include a glossary of all the key vocab. Are you a pup, a pig or a polar bear, for example?* And who got a horny zoologist to name them? It would also feature answers to queer FAQs like: Which holiday destinations are most likely to murder you because of your sexual orientation? Upon introducing your new other half, when do you go for 'boyfriend' or 'partner', and when do you pull out the 'fuck-puppet'? If someone says, 'Which of you is the man in the relationship?' is it OK to chin them? Can you really be gay if you get on with neither the music of Lady Gaga nor your own mother? A more advanced edition a few years down the line might explain the appeal of Liza Minnelli and – crucially – include a lot of information concerning the ins and outs of gay marriage, with a full chapter on proposing, and how the fuck that works.

J and I had been together seven years and I'd spent half of

---

* A pup wears a neoprene snout and gets hauled around on a lead; a pig is unafraid of fists, urine or faeces finding their way into the bedroom and a polar bear is a white-haired older man with a substantial chassis. Saves you googling it and getting served kink-based ads for the next twenty years.

it wondering whether I should propose. I knew I wanted to get married, I just needed to be sure I was asking for the right reasons: because there was nobody else for me, because the two of us made sense when nothing else did, because it would show my lifelong commitment to our love.

But it always felt like there was room for doubt. Was I chasing a feeling I used to have – the married doctor: reliable, respectable, the cult of normality? Essentially, was I just dragging J into my personal psychodrama?

I did this multiple choice in my head most days and eventually arrived at the answer. We were happy, secure, stable and sharing a life and a mortgage. I definitely wanted to be married to J, I felt I had grounds to propose and I was over 80 per cent sure he'd say yes. Plus it would generate a tax saving of £240 per annum and really annoy my parents. I knew when it needed to happen (on his birthday, to pull focus and make it more about me) but the *how* seemed almost prohibitively complicated.

Much like everything in life, the rituals around proposing are set up in a very heteronormative way. Traditionally, the man buys the woman as disgusting and ostentatious a diamond ring as he can afford, which the woman instantly compares to her friends' rings and realises she should have married that banker she secretly sucked off at Jessica's party. Then on their wedding day, they can only exchange simple wedding bands because they've just spent all their money on the 'bronze package' at what's described in the brochure as a country house hotel, but which actually has the atmosphere of a Soviet labour camp.

I took myself off to Bond Street. I'd have preferred Argos but the only time I remembered J being remotely positive about a piece of jewellery it was not from Argos. Alas, it was a Cartier bangle, so I thought that was a decent if madly overpriced bet. This is definitely a purchase you don't want to fuck up.

I told the man at the shop that I was intending to propose and he pointed me towards an array of solitaire diamonds. I explained the concept of homosexuality and was informed that the usual protocol for the homosexual gentleman would be for 'Sir' to buy a *pair* of identical rings from him, at once, at huge expense. Then we would have matching rings, which was apparently very important, and would give me something to commemorate the proposal, other than a doubly depleted bank account. I mean, of course he'd say that, but it did make sense for me to get both rings out of the way at once. I am, after all, still waiting for J to frame my degree certificate like he promised to nearly a decade ago, so it made sense not to rely on him to suddenly get his shit together.

And what about the wedding day itself? Apparently, at this point Sir would traditionally buy a matching pair of Cartier watches to mark the occasion. Would he fucking now?

Anyway, as I was there, I thought I might as well see what was on offer. Sir was brought a plump cushion of gaudy, flamboyant rainbow-bejewelled rings that even Elton would consider a bit ostentatious. But given they started at twenty grand, my opinion of them was fairly moot. I asked to see a plainer selection, hoping that this would bring the asking price down by a couple of digits. Happily, it did.

The cheapest ring that Cartier sold was not only tasteful and almost affordable but it also had a lovely personal connection to me, so I handed over my card, asked for a pair of said rings to be boxed up, and waited for the inevitable anti-fraud call from the bank. It's what's known as a Russian ring. Not because it contains an ornate golden egg or dispenses polonium but because it's made to a Russian design composed of three interlocked rings, traditionally in three different colours of gold. The three rings presumably have some kind of meaning; the Holy Trinity perhaps, or maybe the Musketeers or Rod, Jane and Freddy. The rings slide pleasingly, almost seductively, back and forth over each other, which has since become a therapeutic, almost addictive pastime during tedious meetings.

Which brings me to the personal connection. I first saw a Russian ring during my stint as a urology house officer, when a man in his thirties had decided to replicate the pleasing sliding feeling one feels around one's finger, around his penis. Naturally.

Now, if a person is to place a ring designed for their third-fattest finger onto their penis, then the penis in question must be flaccid. (Except in the most heart-rending of cases.) Not pausing to consider the effect of a pleasant sliding feeling on the diameter and density of his penis, or indeed the inelastic properties of gold, the man found himself in considerable pain. You might think that in this situation, a penis would think, 'Fuck this – time to retreat.' But fluid dynamics were not on its side. With no way for the blood to drain out of its engorged shaft, the poor chap's penis slow danced across the Dulux chart from a robust red to a dramatic purply-black. Only then came his acceptance that it probably wasn't going to resolve itself on its own, so he took the inevitable trip to A&E.

DIY cock rings are one of the standard panoply of A&E admissions. There's even a special name: penile incarceration. The object may vary – a wedding ring here, a curtain ring or a wingnut there – but for the doctor, the treatment is always the same: cut it off as quickly as possible,* then tell everyone about

---

*   The ring, not the penis.

it for the foreseeable future. With a Russian ring, of course, the penis isn't free until all three rings have been cut, and so the A&E registrar was happy to let me have a bash at one of them. It was like emancipating a leech. The man was left with a brutalised penis and a wedding ring cut into six pieces, both matters that would presumably take a fair deal of explaining to his wife.

J said 'sure' to my proposal, and I asked him to say 'yes' instead, because I wasn't prepared to organise a wedding on the basis of a 'sure'. In the end, we opted for the least-possible-hassle model: a register office with strangers. This made the most sense to us because we've never exactly been the kind to go in for big public displays of affection – an 'x' at the end of a Christmas card is pushing it. Then there's the fact that all weddings are basically awful. People don't like to be reminded of this; it's the elephant in the white dress in the room. There's nothing enjoyable about sitting in an arctic church where a mystery child won't stop shrieking; or endless photos; or killing time for five hours before eating some withered chicken supreme at such an unnatural time that it puts you out of kilter for a few days, like culinary jet lag; or wincing through speeches that are far too long (most), borderline racist (father of the bride) or written by someone else (every City boy circa 2013); or specially learned dance routines; or swaying along to a band that the groom heard at a function and thought were amazing but he must have been incapacitated by psilocybins at the time because they actually sound like five cats taking each other apart with chainsaws.

But also, and probably most importantly, I'd already gone down the 'proper' wedding route. I'd joke that it was because half of the guests had heard my wedding speech before but the truth is, I lost almost all of them in the divorce. Initially, I thought they sided against me because I blew up the marriage and was therefore the most culpable. But I came to realise that, true as that was, I was also the much less likeable of the two of us.

Meanwhile, J felt that a big wedding wasn't the route he wanted either. I initially assumed he was worried about everyone he knew and loved being in the same place in case the International Space Station crash-landed on the venue. But then I twigged there were other forces at play. It was written in his eyes, across his forehead and, perhaps most crucially, in a text message conversation he was having with his friend MJ, which Apple, for reasons known only to Steve Apple, decided to also send to the iPad I was using at the time. He wanted it to be his big day, not my encore, which was fair enough.

And so we married at a register office in Hammersmith, with two strangers as witnesses – like in a film. Except, rather than two charmingly eccentric and delighted passers-by, we had a pair of council workers from the next office down, who were palpably irritated by yet another happy couple who hadn't thought through the day's logistics and were consequently ruining their lunchbreak.

'Oh, you speak English!' said the registrar.

'Do most people not?' I asked, suddenly concerned that we were about to be conjoined in unholy matrimony by Nigel Farage, a hair-trigger away from a speech about bloody foreigners, coming here and taking our rites of passage. 'No, it's just you've gone for the vows that people normally choose because they can't speak much English. Well, any English.'

J thought we were keeping things simple but on reflection they were a little bit 'Me Tarzan, You Jane'.

The registrar got to work filling out the certificate that I would manage to lose on the District Line twenty minutes later. He asked us to confirm the spelling of our names★ and our addresses. Then occupations.

'Television producer.'

'Writer.'

'You didn't even pause,' said J afterwards. 'You normally have to stop yourself before saying doctor.'

Maybe that was the biggest change of all. I was free. And all it took was a kiss.†

★ One final must-have chapter for the gay starter pack concerns the protocol over surnames. Most people seem to go down the hyphen route. It makes you appear very, very posh for one thing, which no one wants – a bit like if you had an eye operation that meant you had to permanently wear a monocle. And has anyone worked out what happens in a few generations' time when all the double-barrelled kids have kids of their own and every single person on earth sounds like a firm of solicitors?

Then there's the 'live, laugh, love' version where you cut and shut two surnames together – Robinson and White, say – to create a new name, like Robinshite. Or presumably we could just choose something brand new that we both like? Would my publishers mind if my future books had 'Adam Sparklehorse' on the cover?

† And several years of self-doubt, overthinking and soul-searching.

Chapter 24

Medicine serves you a lot more sticks than it does carrots – you'll be dragged over the coals for something you've fucked up a hundred times more than you'll get a pat on the back. Perhaps that's what led me to performing on stage. A theatre full (or quarter full) of people clapping and telling me I've done a good job is a whole lot better than being called into a three-chair disciplinary meeting because I wrote some notes in blue ink instead of black.

But like a toddler who's demolished a grab bag of Haribo or a twenty-two-year-old hospitality worker after their first gumful of MDMA, the highs of performing are always followed by a sudden crashing back to earth – a four-hour drive home or the umpteenth consecutive night in a service station hotel where the only forms of entertainment available are a vending machine, ITV2 or dogging. Maybe there *is* something to be said for never being praised in the first place.

In Glasgow, I came off stage to a middle-aged woman taking a shit in my dressing room.* On the plus side, she was shitting in the toilet, as opposed to on the floor, in the sink or in the

---

* Not regularly, I should add. It's not my super-weird rider: a vaseful of black tulips, 500g of Werther's Originals and a middle-aged woman taking a shit.

breast pocket of my jacket. On the downside, there was still a middle-aged woman taking a shit in my dressing room. And she'd left the door wide open.

'Oh, I'm sorry!' I said instinctively, assuming I'd walked into the wrong room. Backstage areas are notoriously indistinguishable, like the endless identical corridors in a game of Doom. Having said that, it would have to be a *very* similar dressing room, right down to the unmistakeable cumstain on the sofa that meant I'd spent my pre-show hour standing up. (Avoiding the stain, I should say, rather than taking an hour to create it.) Nope – that was my sweatshirt hanging up. This was definitely my dressing room. There was definitely someone shitting in my dressing room.

I stood outside in the hallway, stage-sweaty and in need of a careful-around-the-cumstain sit down and a tall glass of water, and I attempted to rationalise matters. She was a member of staff, surely. She was a kind and cheery member of the crew who worked so hard to make the magic of theatre happen, who had suddenly and irreversibly been caught short. Probably the microwaved mini quiche she'd eaten in the staff room. I was sure she'd be done soon (it had been a while now), at which point I'd hear an embarrassed flushing, a rushed hand-rinse, and watch her slink past me, whispering a quick 'so sorry' as she went to go and re-stock the blue roll or change the fuse in a speaker. I looked at the posters on the wall – all the big names who had trod these same boards before me. What would Noel Edmonds have done in this situation?

'Do you, uh, work here?' I eventually shouted through the dressing room door. Her response was so slurred and unintelligible that if it did turn out to be a yes, someone should probably have a word with HR. I scuttled back to the side of the stage and asked Drax if he wouldn't mind popping into my dressing room and having a quick word with the person who was in there, shitting. Drax's role on the tour involved carrying all the heavy stuff out of the van – if push came to shove, I'm pretty sure he could also carry the van itself – so he felt like a sensible person to manage the shituation.

Drax went in and the interloper explained that she'd simply got lost and hadn't realised it was my dressing room. Not 100 per cent convincing, as the door did have a fairly unmissable sign with my name on it. But no harm done, foetid stench aside ('Can someone find the big thing of Febreze!?'). The Slurring Shitter seemed harmless and hammered enough to be innocent of any crime beyond dropping a torpedo into my VIP U-bend, so she was sent off home.

Only then did I notice that . . . things had gone missing. Quite a lot of booze, for a start. In the relatively short length of time my show took, she'd smashed her way clean through a bottle and a half of Oyster Bay, although the toothmarks on the caps of the beer bottles implied that wine wasn't her first choice. My Cadbury's Fingers had also been obliterated, along with both packets of Monster Munch.★

My working diagnosis was therefore that the intruder had left mid-show to look for the toilet, had become radically lost and found herself backstage. Intrigued by what my dressing room might look like, she'd opened the door a crack and was delighted to find not three bowls of porridge and three empty beds but a treasure trove of mid-priced supermarket wine and a selection of tuck shop snacks. So she got to work eating

---

★ I'll concede my rider is less 'rock and roll band who makes a groupie have sex with a fish' and more 'drunk man buys dinner from an overlit corner shop', but who wouldn't want a few paws of Monster Munch after a gig?

and drinking, and by the time she dropped the abducted kids off at my pool, it was the end of the show, and that's where we met.

Drax ran in excitedly – there had been a development. The venue staff had been clearing out the auditorium when they found one of my dressing room's wine glasses by a seat. So my less generous final explanation for what had happened was that Glasgow Goldilocks had found her way to my dressing room, taken a glass of stolen wine back to her seat, then watched a bit of the show and thought . . . nah, fuck this shite. There's fucking Monster Munch back there.

I was lying on the bed in my Premier Inn* that evening and dreading the morning's drive from Glasgow to Hove (was this tour booked in alphabetical order rather than by consulting a map?) when J rang. 'How was the gig?'

I told him exactly how it went, in full scatological detail. Even though I was hundreds of miles away and I didn't see him much more than I would if I was working on a labour ward, I was now doing a job where I could honestly say how my day went, rather than just brave-facing it and saying, 'Fine, thanks.' But ultimately, it was a job where a bad day is never going to be a catastrophe – a baby doesn't die, a Glaswegian lady simply defecates in your dressing room.

'Oh well, at least you know the tour's already hit its low point,' said J. 'That's got to be the worst thing to happen to you at a gig?'

Hell, no. It was barely the worst thing to happen to me at a gig that year. For example, the fox-hunting charity gig I'd

---

* 'Everything's Premier but the price, and the room.'

been booked to speak at, which on arrival, turned out to be a *pro* fox-hunting event.*

And there was Sheffield – I got back to my dressing room at the interval and the place had been ransacked. My overnight bag was gone and, with it, my house and car keys, my phone, my laptop, my wallet, my passport and a Will Self novel. The implications of replacing all that didn't really bear thinking about (with the exception of the Will Self novel – I have a good charity shop round the corner). My manager, Bruce, was with me at this show and immediately called my phone – it rang and rang before going to voicemail. But at least it was alive – there was hope! I asked him to keep ringing it during the second half in case someone answered and if they did, to offer cash for its safe return.

Meantime, I went back on stage in an understandably foul mood and essentially accused the entire audience of stealing my stuff. As every powerless but well-meaning substitute teacher can attest, 'You're not leaving until someone owns up!' is not the most effective crowd work. But the audience was innocent, so I had to let them go. Not least, by law. Less innocent was the man who eventually answered Bruce's phone calls. Apparently he'd been through my wallet and had been struck by the name, or more specifically by the title, on my bank card: DR ADAM KAY. Immediately, he was remorseful. He couldn't possibly steal from a doctor, he explained. They'd done so much for him, after all. Bruce thought it best not to mention the fact that I'd not worked as a doctor for some years and only really hung onto the title in case it eventually got me an upgrade

---

* To be fair to far-right ghouls, it must be slightly difficult to book comedians for your various extreme functions. There are only so many times you can watch Geoff Norcott and Jim Davidson.

on a plane. Sadly, this scoundrel's interpretation of 'couldn't possibly steal' was decidedly looser than mine, because when my belongings were returned to me, they were short of the cash in my wallet, my leather jacket and – strangely – the Will Self book. What remained, which amounted more or less to my entire life, he valued at a ransom of £60. Even though it saved me a morning on the phone to the bank, a trip to the key cutters and having to re-write the first 20,000 words of a doomed novel,★ it was so derisory as to be a little insulting – if you're going to leverage my earthly belongings for cash, mate, at least make it a three-figure sum.

'So was *that* your worst gig, then?' asked J, as I watched a moth kamikaze itself into the hotel room window over and over.

'Yeah, probably,' I lied.

★ A time-travelling serial killer mystery that was basically a combination of *Silence of the Lambs* and *Goodnight Sweetheart*. If *Time Crime* ever hits the shelves, please think twice before buying it.

– FLASHBACK –

Worst Gig

I had entered the death rattle phase of my medical career. I was doing the job to the best of my ability but the lighthouse was increasingly unmanned. Comedy had always offered me a way out, to stay sane: whether through writing in my diaries, or doing a few stilted turns behind the mic at comedy clubs. It was a release, of sorts. I would also occasionally find myself embroiled in the strange world of 'corporates' – performing in grimly up-lit function suites as part of a company's away day or Regional Salesperson of the Year awards ceremony. Driving back home afterwards with a thin wodge of banknotes in my pocket made me feel almost famous – well, as famous as you can feel with an Esso ploughmans sandwich sliding around the dashboard.

The opportunity arose to perform a twenty-minute set at a medical conference in New Zealand. On the face of it, it wasn't a particularly attractive proposition: they would pay me to fly out, stay one night, perform and zoom straight off stage to the airport. I was welcome to extend my trip as long as I wanted, but I would have to fund that myself using my no savings. So, a day trip to New Zealand it was. But I was pretty confident that my years of working laborious shifts (literally – a quick glimpse at the quality of my material for you there) and stealing naps in uncomfortable chairs meant I'd be totally unfazed by this adventure in deep vein thrombosis and time zones.

H tried to explain that the numbers didn't really make sense. I'd be away from home for five days, travelling for most of it, using up a hunk of my annual leave, and my fee would work out at less than minimum wage as a result. I explained that, yes, it seemed like an endurance test but it could lead to amazing new opportunities. When that went down like a vomit Vichyssoise, I switched to begging, for days and days, like a toddler desperate for a puppy. But I had another motive for making the trip that I'd declined to share: I had decided to cheat on her.

I know what you're thinking. Even now, years after the event, you're willing me to reconsider. But I'd already worked through all this with the perky little devil on my left shoulder and the rather beleaguered little angel on my right.

Reasons this was bad:

1. Cheating is bad.

2. Premeditated cheating is probably worse than spontaneous cheating, in the way that murder is worse than manslaughter.

Reasons this was totally fine:

1. I was going to another hemisphere to do it, so she couldn't possibly find out or get hurt. It was considerate, even.

2. It would only be this one time.

3. I wasn't lusting after anyone in particular, I didn't know who I was going to cheat with, just that it needed to happen. It was hardly like I'd arranged an intercontinental hook-up with her best mate.

4. I would be cheating on her with a man – a possessor of a penis, balls and beard trimmer, so it basically didn't count.

I had already committed to spend the rest of my life with H and I really wanted to do that, but there was a boil that needed lancing, something I had to do one last time, for old time's sake, to finally clear my body of the pathogens. My internet search history for the past six months would have made Freddie Mercury blush and I had decided this was the only way to resolve it. Then it would go away forever and I could move on with my nice, normal straight life. Bottled lager! Formula 1!

The numbers spoke for themselves – only two reasons it was bad, against a massive and very well-argued four reasons it was absolutely fine, if you think about it. Which I did, feverishly, constantly, from the picosecond the gig was offered to me until the moment I touched down. After a full day chewing my nails on noisy, airless, cramped aeroplanes, I creaked into the hotel and my body attempted to unfurl itself.

I was going into all this with my eyes wide open and armed with reams of data about every possible gay venue in the city – bars and clubs, outdoor spaces, saunas – the full gamut from seedy to fabulous. Bars and clubs, I decided, were too public. Even though my own parents had once walked past me on a train platform without spotting me, I was convinced that here in New Zealand I would be instantly rumbled. Somehow, a touring party of everyone me and H had ever met would be sat two tables over from me, and the news I was knocking back margaritas in a bar called Popperz would be immediately relayed back to her. Meeting outside felt decidedly criminal and I was in no mood to leave New Zealand with mugshots and a lifelong ban from returning. Saunas sounded nauseatingly unsanitary but probably the most appealing / least appalling option and the best chance of getting what I wanted pronto and incognito.

The hotel had kindly given me a map of the local area, circling the restaurants that had bribed them the most, and my chosen sauna was at the very edge of it, a fifty-minute walk away. I stared into the grid, its efficiency and sense of order a soothing counterpoint to the chaos and excitement. I used my finger to trace the journey I was about to take. Or maybe I shouldn't? It wasn't too late to alter the timeline – I could just lie in my hotel bed and watch people on gameshows win jackpots in weird currencies. No. It was time. Once opened out, the map refused to fold back into its compact state again, despite upward of twenty attempts, like it was some kind of *Crystal Maze* challenge. Did it have some kind of metal underwiring? Or was the map itself making a last-ditch attempt to stall me? No, it's me who's stalling this time, because I know where this story is going, and I don't need a map.

I walked to the sauna. If I didn't, my brain told me, then any cab I took or bus I rode would be driven by H's cousin's neighbour's cousin's neighbour, and the chain of inevitability would be set in motion. Thanks to my research, I could picture the entrance to the sauna in my head – but I was still a little surprised to come across it for real. I stood for a while around the corner, watching, making sure the coast was clear and that there were no hidden cameras or hunting nets ready to fall on me.

The reception area was small and seemed to be lit by the glow of a Casio watch. A man stood behind a counter, expressionless, neither friendly nor unfriendly, just . . . there. I was expecting him to press a red button and have me arrested but instead he told me the entrance fee, held out his hand for the cash and asked my name. For what, the guest book? 'Brian and Kevin were wonderful hosts – hopefully next visit we'll have time to check out the harnesses!'

I gave a fake name, which I imagine is fairly standard, but spiced things up a little by using an unconvincing French accent. I'd practised this quite a few times in the hotel, like I imagine all the best spies do. There was always a risk that the guy on the front desk would hear my flawless cadences and reply in my newly adopted native language. Luckily he didn't, so I wasn't forced to wheel out the only French I remember: asking for a return ticket to Dieppe and telling him the library is closed. He handed me a locker key on a wristband and a white towel that had definitely spent some time getting to know a grey sock or two in the washing machine, then nodded towards the changing room door.

The locker room was mercifully empty. I stepped gingerly out of my clothes and squeezed the towel around me, its width slightly narrower than my circumference. Off with my watch, on with my wristband, then through to the fuckatorium. I felt sick – not so much butterflies in my stomach as a churning mound of bats.

There was something very odd about walking into a

sauna that had extremely loud music playing – a place of relaxation reimagined to be utterly unrelaxing. Like getting an aromatherapy massage from a masseur who can't stop screaming. Half a dozen men were sat around wearing the same uniform: white towel and wristband – in here, we're all anonymous and equal. I had expected there to be more customers and, while I was glad not many people would see my face, it was also slightly alarming to discover there were only six other people in this city as perverted as me. They looked up and I smiled nonchalantly. Well, I was going for nonchalantly – it could have quite easily been anything from a scowl to a serial-killer grin.

I realised that my research left me in the dark from this point – I was new to the world of saunas, let alone international ones. How does it work? Do we flirt? Am I meant to talk? Where do we go? Surely we don't kiss? What actually happened hadn't occurred to me as a possibility: a man in his forties stood up, took my arm and wordlessly led me to a dimly lit cubicle, where he raped me.

I was brought up well – I like to give people the benefit of the doubt. I've tried to put myself in my rapist's situation again and again, to work out if there could have been some kind of misunderstanding – something I did wrong. I would have preferred that version of events – I could chalk it up to experience and pledge to communicate better next time. But I can't – the truth of it is inescapable. I said no when it became obvious he wanted this interaction to go a lot further than I did. I said no, again, when he started. I said no when he overpowered me and pushed my head into a wipe-clean cushion that stank of antiseptic. The smell took me out of the moment and briefly back to hospital – being transported away was no bad thing.

I tried to scream, knowing even in that moment that I wouldn't be heard – not by this man who didn't want to hear and not by anyone else, thanks to the rhythmic pounding of the music. I soon stopped bothering, concentrating instead on the pulse I could feel in my ears – a reassuring reminder that I was still alive, and something that I could count until it ended. 1 . . . 2 . . . 3 . . . 4 . . . 5 . . . It has always helped me to count – the number of lengths left until I've finished my swim, the number of patients left to see in clinic. 36 . . . 37 . . . 38 . . . 39 . . . And I knew this would end – whether it lasted four seconds or two hours, it had to end eventually.

The inconvenient clarity of hindsight makes me wonder if the fact I stopped saying no and screaming acted as implicit consent. Signalling that he was right to carry on, that I'd just been playing hard to get, that I loved it really, that I was just like all the rest. And there had to be others, didn't there? He was too blasé, too confident to be new to this.

363 . . . 364 . . . 365. Six minutes if my pulse was going at sixty beats per minute. Three, if my pulse was 120, which was probably more likely. He peeled himself away from my body, and muttered 'Thanks', before leaving. Thanks. You don't say thanks to someone you've just raped, do you? Was coming here in the first place my consent? Not pulling my hand away when he took my arm – was that a way of saying yes, in a language I'd never been taught, negating everything I would say afterwards?

There was another man in the locker room when I got back into my clothes. He said hi and I reciprocated. 'Oh, are you from the UK?' Fuck. I'd forgotten my *'Allo 'Allo* impression. I said I was from Hartlepool, even though I didn't and still don't know where that is.

Through reception, then out into the night. I don't remember much about my walk to the hotel – the streets were a slow, blurry trudge. I must've gone the long way round, or stopped to collect whatever thoughts I could, because by the time I got back to the hotel, the reception desk was closed and I had to buzz for the night porter. He looked at me conspiratorially, as if he knew what I'd been up to, and asked me if I'd had a good evening. I found myself saying yes.

Everything I knew about rape came from watching TV dramas: you get straight into the shower and scrub and scrub and scrub yourself clean before sliding hopelessly down the tiles to the floor and sobbing into your bruised knees. But as soon as I started to get undressed, I needed my clothes back on immediately, to shut my skin away – even the air on my flesh repulsed me. I slept in my jeans, shirt and the same blood-stained underwear I'd walked home in. The fabric was my armour, keeping the shame and secrets inside, reality and judgement out.

You hear of people questioning their belief in god after life throws them some appalling roll of the dice. I suddenly questioned my atheism: what other rational explanation could there be for what happened beyond a vengeful deity, furious at my trifecta of sin: infidelity, depravity, dishonesty. Quite the charge sheet for what was barely a stopover.

Contacting the police and putting this nightmare on public record was unthinkable. Saying it out loud would make it real – I would never be able to deny it or pretend it hadn't happened, which already felt like my only way of getting through it. Plus of course it would launch me into a spiral of bureaucracy that would see me miss my gig, delay my flight home and eventually find myself explaining everything to H. She mustn't find out, especially now there was so much to hide. I told myself the case was flimsy anyway – the police, probably puritanical straight men with 2.4 New Zealand children, would tell me you can't get raped if you go somewhere looking specifically for sex. What was I expecting to happen in a place like that – a round of backgammon? And as for the man who attacked me, what were the realistic chances of ever finding him? Did I even want them to find him? What if he told them I was begging for it, putting words into my mouth to fill the silence of my own making? Besides, if I could lie about my name and fake my voice, didn't that make me the most unreliable witness?

And so I lay there staring at the ceiling of my hotel room, acting as police, judge and jury, and coming to the decision that I should somehow just try to move on. Lifting the rug and sweeping everything under it – it was in my doctorly DNA. I don't think I slept, but it was hard to tell – replaying the same sequence in your head a hundred times is pretty similar to a nightmare.

And then I had to make people laugh for money. I've never thought of those two theatre masks as comedy and tragedy, more as how I present myself on stage versus how I actually feel. All I had to do that day was paint the mask on when I left the hotel room rather than when the MC read out my name. The perennial petty frustrations of the soundcheck came as a weird kind of relief. Asking if we could swap the wireless SM58 mic for a wired one meant that I couldn't think about the way the man said 'Thanks'. The high frequency hum from the monitor displaced the thumping sauna music from my head.

I stood in the wings waiting for my spot, as the audience

were treated to incomprehensible PowerPoint presentations about interleukins and epithelial growth factors – it wasn't doing much to warm them up for me but equally well at least I wasn't going to be upstaged by the previous act. I concentrated on the audience rather than the learned lecturers, scanning the room to make sure that my attacker wasn't somehow there. I didn't even know if I'd actually recognise him – shouldn't I be able to remember every line on his face? Was this my brain protecting me or failing me?

And then I heard my name. Time to go on. I've always been proud of my ability to find humour in even the darkest of situations, to plumb the depths of my despair and come up with a laugh – it's how so many medics survive. It's fair to say that here it was pushed to its limits. But if the jokes kept coming, if I could see those eyes smiling and hear the (albeit limited) laughter, I could get through it. For those few minutes, the safe haven of a stage beneath my feet and the lights warming me, I was invincible. The gig went remarkably well, in that I made it to the end without breaking down in tears or announcing that of the five people I'd spoken to in their country before getting on stage, 20 per cent of them had sexually assaulted me. The jokes tumbled out of me on autopilot. I left the same pauses for laughs that I always do, barely noticing or caring whether or not they came. I got my biggest reaction when I told a borderline-decent off-the-cuff joke about the long walk back from the gate being about a quarter of the total plane journey. The fact it landed better than the material I'd been honing for years was fairly grim when I thought about it. Then again, thinking of fairly grim things is a good way of not thinking about extremely grim things.

Contractual obligations fulfilled, I stood outside the hotel waiting for my ride back to the airport – irritatingly, this was in direct view of the conference's drinks reception on the lawn. There's a definite awkwardness to the transition from professional-ish entertainer on stage to scruffy bloke holding a suitcase and looking for a silver Prius. A bunch of audience members spotted me and made their way over to say that I was great, which wasn't technically true but was nonetheless appreciated.* No one could believe I was heading straight home and they all told me how ludicrous this whole trip was. You've got no idea, cobber.

I ordered an Asahi on the plane – a large one. A few minutes later, instead of the frosty bottle of lager-anaesthetic I was expecting, a significant quantity of sake arrived. Embarrassment forced me to drink it all, despite the fact it was repulsive. I should have said something but I couldn't: I'm British, I'm a Kay, I'm a doctor.

H saw me in the kitchen and hugged me. I needed that hug, even though I didn't deserve it. My emotions were almost impossible to process. Relieved to be home, bursting with shame. Knowing I was holding in a secret I couldn't possibly share, terrified that it was written across my face. But more than that, a strange feeling I wasn't quite me – I'd left something behind in New Zealand and come home in an Adam-shaped body that didn't quite fit.

She told me that I stank. I reminded her of my twenty-four hours of air travel, glossing over the fact I hadn't been able to see myself naked for the thirty-six hours before

---

* I'm not sure an audience of Brits would ever do this – I guess New Zealanders are just a lot less reserved and probably that bit nicer. (Although, admittedly, one did bring the average down.)

that. The hygiene situation felt unsustainable, so I had a bubble bath. Something that used to be a Sunday treat was now the only way I could get clean without looking at my body – protected by an opaque foam, letting the water lift off the dirt without having to touch my own skin.

No time for emotions. First on the list: getting tested and retested at a GUM clinic. I almost used my fake name and French accent again, but my alter ego hadn't been much of a good luck charm so far and I needed as much luck as I could get. I was pretty convinced a positive test result was on its way. After all, why should this furious god be done teaching me a lesson when he still had such a good card to play? I didn't have sex with H for weeks, until I'd had the all-clear from the clinic. It was especially painful to push away affection that I needed so acutely – I think she probably thought I was depressed.

I wasn't depressed. I didn't feel angry, or anxious, or worthless, or any of the other things I had always assumed someone who'd been assaulted would feel. The most over-whelming emotion was guilt, a feeling that I was the bad guy. Well, I was the bad guy. It just so happened there was an even badder guy half a world away. I don't think I'd ever known the true meaning of loneliness until then: I was paralysed by it, locked in a soundproof cage. I couldn't think of any other person I could confide in. Who could I trust to under-react, to hide their shock, or be sympathetic and non-judgemental? There would be so much to unpick that it would totally redefine our relationship. How pitiful to have gone this long on the planet and not have a single person I could be totally honest with.

Time is actually a pretty ropey healer. If I was that slow at trying to make people better on the wards, I'd have been struck off by the GMC in week one. But to give time a bit of credit, ten years later is better than two years later is better than six months later is better than two weeks. Thirteen years on and I no longer even think of it when I'm on stage. Mostly.

I didn't tell another human being for over a decade. Even my diary, my confidant for years, was left out of the loop. The sole entries from that trip were my joke about the walk from the gate at the airport and the misunderstanding about Asahi. Maybe I was too ashamed. Maybe I couldn't face the risk that someone would find my diary and read it. Or maybe I just knew from the moment it happened that I would never forget it: every minute, every second, already etched into me in indelible ink, with me forever.

Chapter 25

I took a photo of the bizarre blisters that had been spreading across the palms of my hands for the last few days. I felt like I should probably do something about it when picking up a shopping basket led to bubblewrappish popping sounds and drops of thin fluid, which caused a minor environmental hazard in the entrance to Waitrose.

I spent a good day wondering who was the best person to send my snap – I didn't know any dermatologists, so probably a GP? I was flicking through my contacts list, working out which of my GP mates was least likely to forward the picture around a WhatsApp group, when an outlandish thought occurred to me.

I could . . . see my own GP? They *might* tell me I was over-worrying, or make fun of me, or make me feel bad for not knowing what was wrong with me, or say I was wasting their time. But realistically, they'd be too nice/knackered for any of that so they'd just hand out a diagnosis and pack me on my way. That's what normal people do when they have a medical issue, right?

'Which doctor do you normally see?' asked the receptionist when I called.

Now there's a good question – what was the old boy called?

Ah, that's right. 'Dr Strange,' I replied.

'Oh goodness. Well, I'm sorry to say that he passed away. A few years ago now, actually.'

When I put my jacket on and told J that I was off to see the doctor, he reacted with delighted astonishment, as if I'd found the Koh-i-Noor in the washing basket, or how my parents would if I said I'd gone back to medicine.*

'You're going to the doctor? Not just someone you know? Your actual GP?' I caught him weighing up whether to ask me any more questions, like I was a deer he didn't want to spook. He told me he was proud of me and asked if I wanted him to come along. I reminded him I was going to the doctor with hand blisters, not some terminal diagnosis.

My new GP, Dr Xavier, was extremely nice. He shrugged his shoulders slightly and said he'd refer me to a dermatologist, but meantime handed me a prescription and suggested that I slather on a steroid cream, to see if that helped.† Thirty seconds. Done.

'Is there anything else?' he asked.

---

* Or a wolf if it smelled a – no? OK.

† The dermatologist prescribed me a slightly different steroid, which cleared it up. It was a weird hand eczema called pompholyx, which curiosity is going to lead you to google images of, whether I warn you against it or not. I received a copy of his letter to my GP and scanned it for the all-important first line: the encrypted message about what they think of you. Now that I'm out of the magic circle, I'm prepared to break that code.

'Thank you for referring this pleasant lady/gentleman' – normal patient.

'Thank you for referring this very pleasant lady/gentleman' – nice patient.

'Thank you for referring this extremely pleasant lady/gentleman' – patient sent a thank you card or a bottle of wine.

'Thank you for referring this lady/gentleman' – actively unpleasant patient.

'Thank you for referring this chatty lady/gentleman' – this will be a double-length appointment.

'Thank you for referring this anxious lady/gentleman' – this will be a triple-length appointment.

'Nope! All good!' He'll be glad to have a bit of time to grab a cup of tea or catch up on some paperwork.

I stood up and walked to the door. What an excellent patient I was.

Then I paused. It had taken me god knows how many years to walk through this door, how many more would it take for me to come back? Columbo-style, I told him there was one more thing. I didn't turn round – it felt easier not to look him in the eye. I heard him very gently set whatever he'd been holding back down on his desk. 'Of course.'

I put my hand on the door handle, just in case I changed my mind. Opening up was something I'd always done to someone else, with a scalpel. I needed to be more like J, always so good at telling me what he was feeling, distilling his thoughts into words.

'I don't have a great relationship with food. And I think I might have some kind of PTSD from my old job.'

I heard him take a breath but he didn't say a word. He knew there was something else coming. And so did I. The words came out in tense, heaving staccato. 'And I was sexually as-saulted.'

And then I started crying, and he told me I should sit down to talk this all through.

***

The letter in my hands started with the words: 'Thank you for referring this apparently well-regarded author.' Never read your own reviews.

Chapter 26

In a life that's had its fair share of whiplash moments, one of the oddest turns has been finding myself somehow in the orbit of people who spend their lives being bundled in and out of blacked-out Range Rovers. People who can only eat out at restaurants with private areas to avoid their dinners turning into an endless conga-line of selfie-seekers. People who've become public property. Fame is the unfortunate but inevitable side effect of any kind of success – I'm very much Pluto to their Jupiter/Mickey, but it's fascinating and slightly terrifying to watch.

Having previously done a job that took over every single aspect of my life, I've been extremely keen that this doesn't happen to me again in a slightly different way. I've chiefly managed to achieve this by being nowhere near successful enough for it to become an issue. If I'm ever spotted in the wild, it's almost invariably because a library-dwelling super-recogniser has identified me on the basis of a ten-year-old, Opal Fruit-sized, black-and-white author photo from the back of one of my books.* This happens roughly

---

* Giving a talk to some kids about my book *Kay's Anatomy*, the Q&A session at the end bounced between the usual topics of poo, snot and vomit. Last question – front row, Iron Man jumper, face of an angel. 'Hi Mr Adam. Why do you look so much older than the photo of you in the back of your book?'

once a month, which I think is a fair taxation on the luck I've had.

I tend to avoid TV appearances because they can radically increase the frequency of being accosted in Ryman's. For me, the downsides of featuring on a panel show far outweigh the appearance fee and the opportunity to sit between Josh Widdicombe and Romesh Ranganathan for two hours and pretend to make spontaneous jokes, despite having been sent the topics to prepare three days earlier.★

I have to break my own rule whenever I have a new book coming out, though, because publishers insist on a decent slug of publicity to minimise the percentage of copies being turned into garden mulch. Most of the publicity will be breakfast-sofa-based chat rather than panel shows, which is good, because that means – unless I say something disastrous and become immortalised in a *TV's Most Epic Fails* clip show – my appearance will quickly disappear. It's not like there's a channel called Maeve showing repeats of *Lorraine* and *GMB* every evening until the sun explodes.

But, like panel shows, these ones still have a tiny element of cheating, known as the 'researcher chat'. This is a half an hour phone call where the interviewee gets a handy heads-up about the questions they'll have chucked at them on camera. It's also an excellent opportunity for the production company to find out whether there's any chance at all that the interviewee is an absolute headcase who'll get the TV station taken off air because of some extreme rant about immigrants.

Because I had a new book out, I was on my fifth researcher chat for my fifth TV show. 'And why did you leave medicine?'

★ I realise this is the 'Santa Claus' bombshell for middle-aged men. I'm sorry you had to find out this way.

'And do you miss it?' 'And do you think you'd ever go back?' 'And why did you start writing?' So far, so tedious.

'And do you think you'll ever have children yourself?' I flinched. This felt strangely intrusive – somewhere beyond the level of public property I'm happy for my life to become. Was I being overly sensitive? I did the maths in my head. Was any question fair game if they were allowing me to come on their TV show? Surely not – I wouldn't let them quiz me on my cock size or how long it takes me to orgasm.* In the final analysis, I just didn't feel comfortable with the question.

'Would you ask this question if I were a woman?!' I shot back.

'Umm, yeah, probably?' replied the researcher.

They probably would actually – this is daytime telly after all. But that still didn't mean I had to feel comfortable about it. So I politely explained that I wouldn't be appearing on their show the next day after all, although they would probably describe this move as a strop.

I walked – OK, fine, stropped – into the living room and immediately told J about this ridiculous overreach into my private life, only to be greeted by a crashing silence instead of his undying support and abject indignation. I frequently accuse J of siding against me. ('Maybe they had a reason to steal your phone, Adam? What if they had to call their terminally ill mother? What if they needed to sell it to buy baby formula?') But on this issue, I was absolutely certain he'd have been on Team Adam. Instead, Dr Freud leaned back in his chair and slowly brought the tips of his fingers and thumbs together in front of his face. 'And why do you suppose this makes you so upset?' he wondered.

---

* Longer than you'd think, in answer to one or the other.

I was pretty sure I wanted kids. If life had played out differently, I would already have a twelve-year-old. We'd talked about having kids dozens of times. He sent me articles about the various different routes available for two men who love each other very much, each generally accompanied with a note saying, 'Well, this looks like a fucking nightmare.' The only option that didn't require hellish logistics, several years of planning and the huge altruism of others was child-napping, and even that wasn't without its potential pitfalls. How homophobic of god − all it takes for the straights is a five-minute drunken pump 'n' squirt in a Morrisons car park.

The reason I reacted so badly to the phone call was that it lit up something I'd been burying: that I was probably never going to have the children I wanted. I was forty, with a heart hollower than the north transept of Durham cathedral. I didn't particularly like the idea of being one of those dads who was too old to play football with their kids.* Worse still, what if I just keeled over and died on them when they were still young? Or even if not directly on them, dying near them is still pretty bad. What kind of start in life is that? And say I do hit some kind of traditional life expectancy, I'd still be long dead before the kid was my age now − grief on top of mid-life crisis. This poor child is already fucked and it doesn't even exist.

All of this, of course, supposed that a baby immediately materialised in front of us, which clearly isn't how this stuff works.† Aside from the practical considerations of achieving a pregnancy in the first place, both my job and personal experience has taught me that not everything goes to plan. No

---

* 'Well, I definitely don't believe that you'd *play* football,' said my friend Justin.

† Unless you go for the child-napping option.

wonder it's a process that we'd already dipped our toes into then abandoned more times than *Mad Men.*

'Right,' said J. 'Kettle on, mobile phones away – let's talk this through.' Different coloured pens were produced, Post-its went up on walls. There was a determination in his eyes, an executive confidence – I was getting a glimpse into the skillset of the producer of some of the UK's least successful TV shows. So – what are the pros and cons of having children?

On all pragmatic levels, children are almost exclusively cons. They spell the end of lie-ins, holidays and nights out. They require mucking out, constant attention and enormous unremitting expense. And on the basis of other parents we know, your personality immediately and entirely disintegrates until your once-celebrated conversational pizazz is reduced to wittering on interminably about your offspring. You lose rational perspective, describing your child as a genius after they manage to daub a handprint on a piece of paper, or successfully (although let's be frank, very approximately) imitate the noise of a cow. Plus the world is hurtling hellward in almost every respect, so you're subjecting your child, who you love more than anyone else in the universe and wish a life better than yours, to a future where the only certainty is that it's going to be much, much worse.

The pros are quite nebulous and don't reflect particularly well on you when written down. The joy that they bring you as soon as you make eye contact is quite a big one but it's a slightly selfish arrangement. The idea of passing down your DNA so that you achieve immortality of your genetic material on earth is award-winningly arrogant, and the kind of thing you'd expect from comic book villains or people who lock other people up in cellars. The notion that I'd be a 'good dad' was a nice idea but it wasn't necessarily true.

And also, so what? I'd probably make a decent postman but that didn't mean I should devote myself to 5 a.m. starts and and getting savaged by Cockapoos. To have someone to care for you when you deteriorate into a bed-shaped mess or to supply a selection of compatible solid organs when yours give up the ghost is honest, but not necessarily in the spirit of things.

But then again, so much human behaviour would seem like a very bad idea if boiled down to a list of pros and cons. Getting married, for example. Gym membership. The government. A quick drink after work. But despite what medicine may have taught me, not everything can come down to a logical list of benefits and risks. It's all outweighed by a strange intangible – call it love if you want, call it your brainstem, call it a primal urge – but it's big and it's unknowable and it's real. I wanted to have kids, and J felt the same.

J nervously handed over to me for the science bit. I explained that it obviously depended which route we took, but if we were even considering having kids which were genetically ours, then the first step would be to see if we had sperm which were up to the task. 'We might as well get it frozen at the same time to save money,' I added. J asked why it would cost money, and I said that gay fertility wasn't really covered on the NHS, so he asked if that was homophobic, and I said it probably was, so he asked if we should sue the NHS, and I said that's probably the last thing we should do and googled some private fertility clinics.

We booked in to make our deposits and J marked it in the diary as 'spunk clinic', forgetting that my agent also has access to the calendar.

There's a surprising amount of paperwork involved with jizzing into a cup. One of the forms asked the question of what should happen to our sperm samples if we died. J said that he wanted his to be stored in the freezer, for me to use in the future should I want his children. I said that I wanted mine poured down Chris Hemsworth's throat but the nurse wasn't happy with this answer, so I just copied J's.

And then into the clinic room: a lot fancier than the NHS ones I'd sent patients off to in my fertility days. Rather than a blue plastic waiting room chair, there was a swish red sofa in wipe-clean pleather. And rather than a stack of Caxton-era magazines, the internet. J went into the room next door.

'You've got twenty minutes,' said the receptionist. It's pretty stressful being told that you have to ejaculate within a certain period of time. Whether you're a bewildered sperm donor or a pre-fluffed pornstar, imposing a deadline of any description is never conducive to a nice, relaxed orgasm. Neither was the thought of how many other men had used the same wank-booth. I noticed that a poster informing guests to put their completed samples in the lockable cabinet was dated March 2005. Yikes. Let's say a sample every twenty minutes each working day, five days a week for sixteen years – that's got to be close to a hundred thousand ejaculations in this room. A hundred thousand men, all jerking away on the same couch, all ejaculating in a room the size of a lift. I briefly wondered what a blacklight would reveal, but the resultant mental image wasn't particularly conducive to a rapid orgasm (not personally, anyway – you do you), then I became the 100,001st person to pull down their CKs.

I clicked the remote control's 'on' button – it was linked to internet pornucopia PornHub, which was a relief: it meant at least I could find something to my taste and hopefully get this over with, within the allotted time. As it happened, some quite niche porn was already playing when the screen blinked to life. I watched for a moment as a five-foot skeletal twink (Alejandro, according to the description) was being jackhammered by a much older, seven-foot hairy wardrobe of a man (Gonzalo). It was somehow nice that my predecessor in the room was gay but also unnerving that the telly doesn't reset to some homepage once you're done. I made a mental note to manually close the video when I was done. As Alejandro and his dad were about as likely to do the job for me as an episode of *Bargain Hunt*, I grabbed the remote and started pressing buttons.

No dice. I imagine the insides of the remote control were irredeemably gunked up by hundreds of poorly aimed emissions, amounting to untold quadrillions of doomed, wayward sperm and almost certainly invalidating Panasonic's normally excellent warranty. I turned the TV off and pulled out my phone – no reception. I heard next door's lock click – J was already finished. Bastard. I checked the time. Fuck, only twelve minutes left. Right – me, Alejandro and Gonzalo would have to sort it out between us. It wasn't going to be easy, but where there's a willy, there's a way – and by looking down when there was a touch too much of Gonzalo's hairy back on display and muting the volume so I wasn't put off by his strange, low wheezing sounds, we got there eventually. Into the locked cabinet it went, just shy of twenty minutes.*

As I left the protein pod, the next jizzer was already waiting outside. The correct protocol here is of course to totally avoid any form of eye contact, which I did, marching straight ahead towards the stairs. Unfortunately this chap hadn't read the protocol. 'Alright,' he said, spunking all over the Geneva

---

* In answer to the earlier question.

Convention. I offered him a weak smile in return. 'I loved your book, by the way. *This Might Hurt?*'

Of course today had to be the day, my once a month. Torn between thanking him, breaking into a sprint and politely correcting him on the title, I obviously plumped for the former. It was only when I was out of the building that I realised I should have actually explained that the remote control was broken when I picked it up . . . But no. Now there will always be a group of people who, if ever my name happens to come up, will think: 'Oh, he's that doctor, right? Friend of mine followed him into a wanking room. Apparently he gets off to weird Little and Large fetish porn.'

I surprised myself with how nervous I was when the lab emailed with our results.

Our samples were OK, although mine contained a lot of 'sediment', which sounds pretty disgusting and probably means that a spider fell in the pot while I was on the sofa. J sat me down to have the next stage of the conversation – should we move ahead, and in which direction?

I suddenly realised the speed of the train I was on and pulled the emergency lever. I found myself saying I wasn't sure, that it wasn't quite the right moment, what with how busy we both were with work. What I didn't say was how panicked I was that I might not be cut out for this.

I would love this child with all my heart but children from loving families can still end up massively fucked up. How could I be sure that some small, apparently insignificant thing I did wouldn't be the source of untold trauma? What if my idea of getting it right was actually getting it all irretrievably wrong? What if they didn't want to learn the saxophone? What if, instead of ending up like their affable, social dad who can walk into any room and have everyone eating out of his hand within minutes, they ended up like their awkward dad, the one who hides behind humour and never really speaks his heart?* How can I teach others how to find peace and joy in this world when my attempt at it has been so shitbad?

J sat down next to me, put his hand over mine, smiled, looked into my eyes and decoded all my insecurities. He told me he understood – it needed to be 100 per cent right for both of us, because there were no rehearsals and no rewind buttons – once we were in this, we were in it forever, and we both had to want it as much as each other.

I definitely want kids, and not just to have someone to dedicate my books to, or to stop my mum banging on about grandchildren. And J will be a fantastic dad, I've got no doubt about that – if only to make our children like him the best. I can learn from my mistakes. I can continue to unlearn what I was taught as a doctor, to be open about my feelings, rather than pushing them away or hiding them behind jokes. I've already switched from one act to another – surely I can manage a third?

But not today. At time of press, our sedimentary spunk is sitting in a freezer compartment, awaiting further instructions. There will be a right time, one day. And what a time we're going to have.

---

* I'll leave you to calculate which one is which.

Afterword

While I was writing this book, I heard that Mike Schachter had died. He hadn't turned up for his seventieth birthday party and was found shortly afterwards. It was devastating, unexpected and, to anyone who'd known him, an almost incomprehensible end to a life that had been dedicated to improving the lives of others, seemingly at the expense of his own.

As I scrolled through the scores of online tributes to this wonderful man, I was brimming with tears and pride reading how he'd helped hundreds of medical students over the decades. The stories were often exact echoes of my own: he'd been the only one to notice they'd been struggling; he'd been the only person who not just offered to help but came good on his promise.

As with so many doctors, though, he was clearly better at helping others than seeking help himself. Or perhaps no one took that metaphorical walk across the canteen to ask him how he was doing. The best you can hope for in life is that you leave behind a legacy that makes this world a better place for someone, somewhere, in whatever small way you can. Mike did that. I hope that some of his students have paid that forward as doctors themselves. I hope that I'm able to do something similar.

But what would I say if, in some unfortunate time machine incident, I found myself the one talking to an eighteen-year-old Adam?* Would I tell him to give medicine a go, say that he was here now so he may as well make the best of it? Or would I encourage him to bail out while he still had a few last shreds of nerve, pick up his saxophone and teach people a new way to drive their neighbours up the wall? Maybe I'd give him a gentle nudge to be a GP like his father, with a few coded warnings that it wouldn't be easy but it might be a slightly less chaotic ride than obs and gynae. Maybe I'd be brutally honest – it's a job that means he'll see some really fucked up stuff be utterly normalised, in a health service kept running by the superhuman efforts of the people who work within it, at incalculable cost to themselves.

Or perhaps all I'd say is that it's OK to change your mind – something that medicine doesn't want to acknowledge, often with huge human costs and consequences.

If you're reading this and you're where I was, living a life that others mapped out for you, or a life that you know deep inside doesn't speak to the real you, then you're allowed to press the reset button. It might not be immediate, but you'll feel the improvement in yourself. The people around you will notice it. Even people you'll never know will have cause to be thankful as you start making positive contributions to society and reduce the chances of picking up a machete and going postal in a branch of Pizza Express.

No job in the world is worth destroying yourself over, even if you work in a brilliant, beautiful place like the NHS. It's OK to take a break or a breather. It's also OK to step away

---

* Other than, 'There's going to be a thing called Tesla – buy shitloads of shares in it,' and, 'Long story short, you're gay and it's fine.'

altogether, if that's the right thing to do. In a world of people telling you not to rock the boat, sometimes you have to fuck the boat. Do it with as much love and tenderness as you can manage, but grab your trunks and start swimming. Only you know what's in your heart – whether it's becoming a caricaturist in Leicester Square, moving to Chad or moving in with Chad. I promise you'll sleep a lot better.

If you're reading this and you relate to my difficulty in opening up, I can't pretend that I'm any kind of poster boy. I'm a work in the earliest stages of progress. But I can say that I've never regretted any of the times that I've been honest with friends, family, professionals, anyone – however scary it felt at the time. Putting parts of this book down on paper has been the hardest thing I've ever done, but I know in my heart I won't regret this either. There's always someone you can speak to – give it a try.

I realise this is a slight longshot, but if you're reading this and you're responsible for training tomorrow's medics, then I'd like to ask you two questions.

Are you choosing the right people to be doctors?

And are you training them the right way?

If the answer to both questions is yes then it's possible you've skim-read this book. If the answer is no then you have the chance to change the lives of a generation of doctors and, with them, a generation of patients.

First do no harm.

Acknowledgments

To James, who I don't deserve.

To my brilliant and endlessly patient agents, Cath Summer-hayes and Jess Cooper.

To the constellation of stars who are Orion: especially my wonderful editor Anna Valentine; World's Funnest CEO™ Katie Espiner; marketing geniuses Maura Wilding, Tom Noble, Leanne Oliver and Lindsay Terrell; the wisest pen in publishing Francesca Main; the eternally calm and brilliant Jamie Coleman; together with Sarah Fortune, Jen Wilson, Esther Waters, Victoria Laws, David Shelley and a hundred others for making this book a joy. (To write, that is, not read.)

To PR super-supremo Dusty Miller.

To sentence-sorcerer Justin Myers and word-wranglers Karl Webster and Joel Golby.

To Emma Lloyd-Jones, thank god for you.

To Bentley for their amazing cars. I mean, I don't have one but surely they'll have to send me one after I've said this?

And, most of all, to my family and friends, who never signed up for this shit.

Credits

Trapeze would like to thank everyone at Orion who worked on the publication of *Undoctored*.

Editorial
Anna Valentine
Francesca Main
James Kay
Jamie Coleman

Management
David Shelley
Katie Espiner

Copy-editor
Liz Marvin

Proofreaders
Chris Stone
Sally Sargeant

Production
Katie Horrocks

Legal
Louise Lambert
Maddie Mogford

Editorial Management
Carina Bryan
Charlie Panayiotou
Claire Boyle
Jane Hughes
Sarah Fortune
Tamara Morriss

Editorial Consultants
Justin Myers
Karl Webster

Contracts
Anne Goddard
Ellie Bowker

Readers and Consultants
Dan Swimer
Joel Golby
Kathryn Wheeler

Audio
Georgina Cutler
Jake Alderson
Paul Stark

Design
Helen Ewing
Joanna Ridley
Nick Shah
Steve Leard
Steve Marking

Finance
Jasdip Nandra
Nick Gibson
Sue Baker
Tom Costello

Inventory
Dan Stevens
Jo Jacobs

Marketing
Lindsay Terrell
Tom Noble

Publicity
Dusty Miller
Leanne Oliver
Maura Wilding

Literary Support Dog
Pippin

Sales
Anna Egelstaff
Dominic Smith
Esther Waters
Frances Doyle
Jen Wilson
Victoria Laws

Operations
Chelsey Clark
Ellie Clegg
Helen Gibbs
Isobel Sheene
Natasha Head
Sharon Willis

Rights
Ayesha Kinley
Barney Duly
Jessica Purdue
Louise Henderson